Riding the Diabetes Rollercoaster

A new approach for health professionals, patients and carers

Helen Cooper
Lecturer,
School of Health Sciences,
University of Liverpool

and

Robert Geyer
Professor of Politics, Complexity and Policy,
Lancaster University

Foreword by
Ian Botham OBE

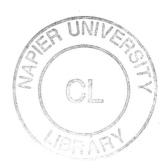
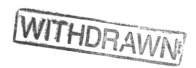

Radcliffe Publishing
Oxford • New York

Radcliffe Publishing Ltd
18 Marcham Road
Abingdon
Oxon OX14 1AA
United Kingdom

www.radcliffe-oxford.com
Electronic catalogue and worldwide online ordering facility.

British Library Cataloguing in Publication Data

A catalogue record for this book is available from the British Library.

ISBN-13: 978 1 84619 045 2

Typeset by Anne Joshua & Associates, Oxford
Printed and bound by TJI Digital, Padstow, Cornwall

Contents

Foreword

Life with diabetes is never easy. My daughter has diabetes and I know that it affects everything she does. In turn, it impacts upon my life and the rest of my family's as well. It complicates our daily routines and it occasionally plays havoc with our emotions. All of this means that a simple, straightforward and trouble-free approach to dealing with diabetes just doesn't exist. Anyone who lives with the disease or cares for someone with it knows this instinctively. Furthermore, health professionals (many of whom I have met through my support for Diabetes UK) often recognise its complexity as well. However, caught within a traditional framework, they have to adhere to a more structured and prescriptive approach that is not always ideal for factoring in individual values, preferences and feelings. This was bought home to me when my daughter, who was diagnosed with diabetes at the age of nine, gained far too much weight at a time in her life (adolescence) when her appearance was extremely important to her. The standard prescription for diabetes at her age is a high-carbohydrate diet. However, as an athlete, I knew that this type of diet would worsen her weight problems (unless she was running marathons!) and undercut her confidence just when she needed it most.

So where does this leave us? Somehow we need to combine the wonderful advances in diabetes treatment with a form of diabetes care that really does recognise the reality of what it is like to live with the condition. The thought-provoking complexity framework in *Riding the Diabetes Rollercoaster* does just that. It questions traditional perspectives on diabetes care for both professionals and people like us, providing both practical tips and thought-provoking ideas. Moreover, it highlights the key part that the patient plays in the self-management of a disease that, at its very heart, is about uncertainties. Such uncertainties need to be recognised and absorbed into our daily lives so that we can play to their strengths. I say strengths because uncertainty means quite simply that you never know when you will 'win.' But with education, training, support and a positive attitude that accepts uncertainty, you may find that every new challenge is a learning opportunity and a chance to grow. These key elements apply to all sportspeople, just as much as they do to the management of diabetes. As *Riding the Diabetes Rollercoaster* states, we are all experts in complexity because that is what makes up our everyday lives. The key is to make the most of it.

Ian Botham OBE
Father of a daughter with type 1 diabetes, supporter of Diabetes UK
and former England Cricket Captain
February 2007

Preface

This book is about choosing a new pair of glasses. For decades, diabetes has been understood, researched and managed through the lenses of a mechanical and orderly set of 'glasses.' These glasses view diabetes as a complicated but knowable condition which can be controlled through patient compliance with health professional advice and health professional conformity to established evidence-based practice. The faith in this particular pair of glasses rests on the fact that it has been around for hundreds of years and has worked in a variety of other areas of human endeavour. Many people therefore continue to assume that these *scientific* glasses are the only ones available. The problem with this, however, is that despite huge amounts of research, funding and effort, diabetes – like many other chronic illnesses – refuses to go away or even to get any easier to deal with. In fact, it is growing enormously, both in terms of the numbers of lives affected and in terms of its physical and human costs. Health professionals have therefore become increasingly frustrated by their inability to develop radical improvements, while patients and carers struggle to comply with complicated self-management regimes.

From the traditional mechanistic and orderly perspective, this is a conundrum. Effort has been and continues to be applied, but the end point remains elusive. The next logical step from this perspective is to change the direction of effort (explore new drugs and therapies) and apply more effort (increase spending and patient compliance) until outcomes improve. But what if . . .?

- What if diabetes is not like a simple mechanical system – for example, a clock – where clear inputs (winding the clock) lead to understandable and predictable outputs (the hands on the clock move)?
- What if the never-ending goal of good blood glucose control is influenced by a complex interaction of evolving factors?
- What if managing diabetes is interwoven into each patient's complex daily life needs and free choices?
- What if health professionals can only know a small part of the true management picture because the evidence/guidelines/reports underpinning practice are so vast that there is just too much to take in and they can never fully know their own patients?
- What if any particular individual's diabetes experience – their self-knowledge – is fundamentally important to outcomes?
- What if diabetes is just part of a larger picture that includes multiple abnormalities accompanying ageing?

How can all of these uncertainties be put into an orderly framework?

The answer is that they can't! Actors looking through the lens of order either have to ignore these questions or keep claiming that more effort and time will solve the problems. The good news is that science, like society, has not stood still, and a different pair of glasses emerged during the twentieth century, known as the complexity framework or perspective. Complexity, emerging out of the physical sciences and rapidly spilling over into the health and social sciences, is a radical departure from the former orderly perspective. It recognises that some aspects of our physical, biological and social worlds are orderly, some are disorderly, and some are a blending of the two, or complex. The key is that rather than try to push everything into an orderly perspective, complexity recognises and embraces the complicated and disorderly nature of our reality.

This may seem absurdly simplistic and 'commonsensical' – everyone knows that things are complicated and complex. And yet, as we hope to show in relation to diabetes, for much of the twentieth century there was a refusal to recognise this inherent complexity and a struggle to make it more orderly. Even today, many health professionals, carers and patients misdirect huge amounts of time and effort in a desperate attempt to 'order' the condition. Patients become passive, rigidly following their doctors' orders to the letter (or not!), rather than recognising the need to balance this professional advice reasonably against their own life priorities. Carers become the health professionals' enforcers, blindly following the old adage that 'doctor knows best.' Health professionals become increasingly frustrated at those patients who won't follow the rules or, to put it more bluntly, 'will not do as they are told.' The problem is that from an orderly perspective there is no way out.

We believe that complexity offers a way forward. It will not cure diabetes. Nor will it solve all of the problems of patients, carers and health professionals. However, by recognising the inherent complexity of diabetes and the human condition and using some of the tools of complexity it can show us that:

- we are all complexity experts even if we don't recognise this
- all of us – patients, carers and health professionals – are experts in diabetes in our own ways
- tensions between patients, carers and health professionals are normal and can be part of a process of creative learning and improved patient self-management
- learning to 'balance' rather than 'control' diabetes is the ultimate goal of diabetes management.

This book is about giving you the opportunity to see diabetes through a pair of complexity 'glasses.' When we began writing the book in 2005, combining Helen's personal and professional expertise in diabetes with Robert's knowledge of complexity, we were confident that complexity was important and that it was a worthwhile perspective for exploring, understanding and managing diabetes. With the completion of the book and the encouraging responses that it has generated, we are confident enough to say that complexity has a real place in the future of diabetes management. As the Nobel Laureate Ilya Prigogine wrote in *The End of Certainty*:

We believe that we are actually at the beginning of a new scientific era. We are observing the birth of a new science that is no longer limited to idealised and simplified situations but reflects the complexity of the real world, a science that views us and our creativity as part of a fundamental trend present at all levels in nature.[1]

So read on and decide which pair of glasses you like best!

Lastly, we would like to thank the Centre for Complexity Research, Lancaster University and the University of Liverpool for their support during the writing of this book. More personally, we would like to thank Samir Rihani for getting the complexity ball rolling, and Jan Bogg and Abbie Badcock for their personal and professional support. Most importantly, we would like to thank our spouses (Kurt and Sigrun) and children (Jessie and Ruth, and Kristoffer and Paul). Without their love and support, this book would have been neither possible nor anywhere near as much fun to write.

Helen Cooper
Robert Geyer
February 2007

Reference

1   Prigogine I. *The End of Certainty: time, chaos and the new laws of nature.* New York: The Free Press; 1997.

About the authors

Dr Helen Cooper

Helen is a lecturer at the School of Health Sciences in the University of Liverpool. She worked for nearly 20 years as a nurse and health visitor, specialising in the field of diabetes before completing her PhD in Liverpool. Her research is centred on patient and inter-professional education and service user participation in training health professionals. She has been an expert adviser to various UK organisations, including the National Institute for Clinical Excellence and Diabetes UK. She has contributed to the UK Diabetes National Service Framework for Retinopathy Screening and Patient Education, and she is a member of the Medical Research Council College of Experts. She has published academic articles in a wide variety of journals and books on diabetes and inter-professional education. In March 2007 Helen won the Diabetes UK 2007 Education Award for outstanding contribution to the evaluation of education in diabetes care. Helen has lived with diabetes for over 40 years.

Professor Robert Geyer

Robert is Professor of Politics, Complexity and Policy at Lancaster University and was Co-Director of the Centre for Complexity Research (CCR) from 2002–2007. He founded the CCR in 2002, has been a Rapporteur on the High-Level Scientific Panel for the EU Framework 6 programme, and has taught at the University of Liverpool, the University of Wisconsin and Marquette University. He has published academic articles in a variety of fields, as well as newspaper articles in Norway, the USA and the UK. His books include (co-edited with J Bogg) *Complexity, Science and Society* (2007), (co-authored with A Mackintosh) *Integrating UK and European Social Policy* (2005), (co-edited with C Ingebritsen and J Moses) *Globalization, Europeanization and the End of Scandinavian Social Democracy?* (2000) *Exploring European Social Policy* (2000) and *The Uncertain Union* (1997).

Introduction

Tony loved football. After he finished school he had to work in his father's shop, but he still managed to play for a local team. His big moment came when his team was picked to play in an FA cup match. They lost 5-1, but Tony scored the one. Pretty soon he got married and when the children arrived, the football was now only on the TV. At the age of 60, Tony retired. At 62 he started coaching at his grandson's football club. It was while he was doing the coaching that the kids joked about his frequent excursions to the toilet. After a trip to his family doctor and some tests he found out that he had type 2 diabetes. Tony was certain that he could 'beat' the disease. He made a list of all the things the doctor said that he could and could not do, when to take the pills, what to eat, how much exercise to take, etc. Tony had always been orderly and methodical at work. It was just a matter of structuring his life to beat the disease. He stopped coaching because it didn't seem to be active enough and it clashed with the timetable he had drawn up. At first things seemed to go quite well, but he began to feel more and more downhearted. He had worked hard all his life and now, when he was finally retired, he was having to work hard again because of this stupid disease. After talking things over with his family doctor and practice nurse, he began to realise that his feelings were commonplace following a diagnosis of diabetes, and he began to move forward in dealing with the complicated emotional side of diabetes. With time he began to realise that he couldn't beat diabetes by work and effort alone. He started relaxing and exploring different ways of living with the disease. He started coaching again. After some unexpected twists and turns his rollercoaster ride was going through a calm stretch.

Jackie is 13 years old. When she was diagnosed with type 1 diabetes at the age of 8 her parents were shocked and she felt scared, but the nurse said that it would be all right, and she liked the nurse. The injections did hurt though, and the hospital smelt funny. The diet wasn't difficult. Her parents were vegetarians so she had always eaten a healthy diet. She was active and could outrun anyone in her class, except Thomas Minford. The problems started when she hit puberty. Her body began to change and keeping the diabetes under control became more and more difficult, and besides she was less interested now. Worse still, she didn't seem to have any 'real' friends. Sure, there was Louise and Rachel, but they just 'acted like children.' She still knew Thomas and wanted him to like her. However, she felt increasingly ugly and fat. She started to decrease her insulin in order to suppress her appetite and lose weight. It worked wonderfully – she lost five pounds in two weeks. Unfortunately, her actions produced another reaction – she lacked energy, was constantly thirsty, her breath smelled and quite soon she collapsed, resulting in a stay in hospital. She couldn't tell her parents what she had done. She knew they wouldn't like it. And what if Thomas found out? She had to get thin or he would never like her. She convinced herself that next time she would be more careful, next time it would be all right. Jackie's ride was at its most difficult and dangerous.

Jennifer is a doctor. She shares a good practice with four other family doctors and sees around 20 to 30 patients a day. She loves and hates her job. She had always wanted to be a doctor, but she hates all of the administration and bureaucracy that come with it. In particular, she hates the continual rule changes that the service managers keep throwing at her and her colleagues. She has many patients with diabetes. Her favourite is Bill, a feisty old man who lives just around the corner from the surgery. For Jennifer, Bill reminds her of her grandfather. The problem is that Bill's diabetes is not responding as it should and she is not sure whether this is due to the disease, or to the way that Bill is managing it. Bill seems to understand the disease and what he has to do, but he is constantly coming to the surgery with various complaints and problems. Bill lives alone, so Jennifer has no way of verifying that he is taking care of himself. Moreover, she thinks that he may be drinking too much alcohol, but she isn't sure. Also, in the back of her mind she is worried that Bill may be inventing symptoms so that he has an excuse to come to the surgery. He may even be inadvertently harming himself in the process. She wishes that she could do more for Bill, but she just can't give him any more time! Other patients are waiting. And is it really right for her to interfere so much in his life? He is an adult, after all. Having spent so much time studying and treating diabetes, Jennifer still finds it terribly frustrating that the diabetes rollercoaster will not go straight.

Peggy and Bob had been married for 30 years before Bob was diagnosed with type 2 diabetes. Bob seemed to take the diagnosis in his stride, but since his initial 'acceptance' Peggy had noticed that he was choosing to ignore the disease, denying it even despite her constant reminders of what he should and shouldn't be doing. He just wouldn't listen to her, and she was feeling more and more frustrated and angry with him. She was frightened for their future – frightened of losing him, or of him going blind, as had happened to his grandmother. She was at a loss about what to do next. As a carer (in this book, the word 'carer' is used loosely to refer to those people who have any level of responsibility towards individuals who have diabetes), her rollercoaster ride seemed to be an endless uphill climb with no clear view of the top.

These are not real stories, but fictional ones that capture general problems of dealing with diabetes. As a patient, it may be the emotional shock and fear, the multiple interacting triggers that cause it to tip into ups (hypers) and downs (hypos), and/or just the dull plod of daily constraints and worries that make it so irritating. For carers and heath professionals, it is also the lack of control and the uncertainty that are so frustrating. In so many areas of medicine there are clear guidelines and procedures to follow. Follow them and the patient's condition should improve. But what can you do when so many factors are involved and the patient's choices and actions are so important. How can you help when so many of these people need more input, but your own work pressures and even the patients won't allow it, or they can't be bothered with the 'rules'?

In many ways, both patients and carers are experiencing the same problem. *The problem isn't diabetes per se – it is the complexity of managing the disease.* In line with western tradition, most of us are determined to view diabetes, and illness in general, as a fundamentally mechanical process. When illness occurs the body is somehow 'broken', like a clock. All it needs is to be 'fixed' and the patient can then return to their previous activities unaltered. The experience of illness is merely a slight or significant deviation from some steady stream of normal life. Many conditions do seem to fit this way of thinking. A simple cold, a broken bone and even some chronic conditions either solve themselves or, with the appropriate tools – a plaster cast on the broken limb or suitable drugs – are easily repaired or restored and the patient resumes normal life.

Diabetes, and many other chronic conditions such as stress, pain and addictions, don't fit this pattern. It is as if try as we might, we just can't get the clock to work. It keeps going too fast or too slow and sometimes breaks down completely. These are diseases of uncertainty. Again, the problem is not the understanding of the disease process – it is our mental picture of the disease and the body as a simple mechanism. If we change our way of thinking we may be able to understand the true nature of living with, working with and/or caring for diabetes, and be better able to manage its individual development as it interweaves itself into the lives of all those involved.

This book is about promoting a new way of thinking. It is not a medical manual for exploring the latest developments in the field. We make no pretensions in that direction. Nor is it a guidebook to help patients with such basics as how to inject, manage weight, exercise, etc. There are many good books to choose from for this, and many which are focused on specialist aspects of the disease and categories of patients (type 1 and type 2 diabetes, young or elderly, and so on). Instead, it provides a broader scientific and philosophical framework for understanding the nature of the disease and its relationship to patients and their development. The name of this new way of thinking is that of a scientific framework called *complexity science*, or just *complexity*.

Strangely enough, although it sounds sophisticated, it is actually rather simple and reflects the everyday life around us. Complexity science emerged out of the growing criticisms of the eighteenth- and nineteenth-century visions of a fundamentally orderly universe and nature of human beings. This earlier framework of order saw the natural world and human beings as basically orderly and, in many ways, mechanical. In this framework, medicine was about fixing the broken bit of the human 'clock.' The hope was that as more and more bits of the clock were understood, any broken bits could be fixed, and eventually there would be no sickness or disease. The dreams of the *Star Trek* generation, where illness was something you studied in historical textbooks, would finally come true!

However, as more and more scientists and thinkers were realising during the twentieth century, nature and human beings are just not that orderly. From Einstein's theory of relativity through studies of species evolution to computer simulations of the weather, it became increasingly obvious that we were surrounded by natural systems that would not follow orderly rules. Similarly, human beings, despite being pressured by horrifically tyrannical totalitarian regimes, refused to follow one developmental pathway (communist, dictatorial, fascist or even pure free market). In medicine, more and more diseases just wouldn't go away, and new ones kept emerging.

Given all of these difficulties, a new framework began to emerge covering a wide range of phenomena, roughly titled *complexity science*. Put most simply, complexity argued that although some natural and human phenomena are basically orderly or disorderly, many are complex combining elements of order and disorder. In other words, in complex phenomena or systems some rules did still fit, but the exact nature of the fit or the actions of the system were not perfectly predictable. One can predict the boundaries of a complex system, but not its exact outcome. Human life is a wonderful example of a complex system. Put someone outside their physical boundaries – say at the bottom of the ocean or in outer space – and they will very quickly and predictably die. But keep them within their physical and biological boundaries, and predicting the exact moment of their death then becomes virtually impossible. For complexity, cause does not always lead to effect, small shifts may lead to massive changes, and totally unpredictable or unknown events can occur even within very simple systems. From this perspective, a degree of unpredictability and uncertainty, and learning and discovery, is not only the mark of reality, but also the sign of a healthy complex system.

To put it plainly, diabetes is a classic example of a complex system. Like all sorts of complex systems that we confront in our daily lives – for example, environmental conditions, traffic systems, work environments, family relationships – they all combine predictable and unpredictable elements into an evolving and emergent whole. In many ways, developing diabetes is no different from any other long-term alteration in our lives, whether it be moving house, the birth of a child, the pursuit of a new career, or the death of a close relative. They all involve managing and balancing new boundaries with the process of making new discoveries and learning. Obviously, no one chooses to have diabetes. But one doesn't choose the death of a spouse or, for that matter, the exact nature of how one's child will develop, or how that development will affect the parent's relationship. All of these systems evolve over time, and attempting to fix the end point of these 'systems' is not only impossible but also frustrating, and can be dangerous.

For the person with diabetes, the problem relates to the dominance of the orderly framework so that the view of diabetes and of him/herself was, and still is for many, fundamentally mechanical. For the patient, it is all a matter of taking the right drug doses, structuring lifestyle as rigidly as possible and hoping for an eventual cure for the disease. Frustration stems from the continual balancing nature of the disease, where even if you do the right thing (with regard to dosages, diet, exercise, etc.), problems and complications may still arise. From an orderly framework, since all problems are basically orderly and you have been told what to do, any mishaps must be the fault of the patient. For the person with diabetes viewing their condition through an orderly lens, guilt can be a frequent companion.

It isn't much better for the carer or health professional in this framework. Steeped in the belief that it is just a matter of effort and control, the carer and professional are condemned to keep quiet or play the role of nagging teachers. Patients should listen and comply if they are to get better. Patients who do not manage their conditions properly are seen as wayward, cheating on their work, not paying attention and not following the rules. For these cases, more monitoring and pressure are necessary to bring out better behaviour. The longer the patient shows a reluctance to self-manage effectively, the greater the pressure that must be applied. Basically, one must make them 'well' despite themselves.

Obviously, this is not true in all cases! Many patients, carers and health professionals refuse to succumb to the pressures that are put upon them, but the pressures remain nonetheless. Over time, it has become increasingly obvious that an orderly framework for diabetes just will not do. In the last 10–15 years the tide has begun to turn. The biggest example of this shift is the transformation in the treatment for diabetes. Rather than treating patients like 'children', researchers have begun to recognise the complex nature of learning how to live with diabetes. Patient education strategies have been developed based on evidence-based guidelines[1] that reflect the importance of self-managing diabetes and of listening to patients, rather than talking at them. Two examples of nationally developed patient education programmes from the UK are

DAFNE (Dose Adjustment For Normal Eating) for type 1 diabetes (www.dafne.uk.com) and DESMOND (Diabetes Education and Self-Management for Ongoing and Newly Diagnosed) for type 2 diabetes (www.desmond-project.org.uk). Patients, carers and health professionals have become partners in diabetes management. This healthy change is not a direct product of complexity thinking, but reflects the general shift away from the orderly framework that is going on throughout the fields of science, medicine and public policy.

We endorse these recent changes, but do they go far enough? Carers and patients are being taught excellent diabetes self-management strategies, but fitting them all together on a day-to-day basis remains a challenge for many. Without a framework to guide this, there will be a natural tendency to drift back towards a more teacher–child type of relationship. This regressive tendency is strengthened by the growing command and control 'accountancy culture' that has emerged in the NHS in the last decade. As increasing pressure is put on carers and health professionals to show results (i.e. meet targets!) for their interventions, they will obviously be encouraged to put more pressure on patients to get these results. And before you know it, we are back to where we started from!

We are certain that the best way to stop such a disaster is to empower those actors at the bottom of the health pyramid – patients, carers, and 'at-the-coalface' health professionals – with not just the right diabetes management strategies, but also the knowledge of a scientific framework that underpins these strategies. With the complexity framework people can begin to develop a very different philosophical approach to self-management – one that focuses on real-world issues, addresses the many different interconnecting parts of a long-term condition like diabetes, and addresses the emergent nature of learning how to live with the condition. In essence, this book takes a first tentative step in bringing the complexity framework down from the world of research institutes and academic departments to the level of those who need it most, the ones who can bring about real and lasting change, namely patients, carers and health professionals.

How are we going to do this? We shall start with a brief introduction to diabetes, outlining some of its main aspects and charting historical developments to show why it is such a perfect example of a complex system. In the following chapter, we shall introduce the reader to the basics of complexity science. Using an historical approach we shall chart the pathway of complexity's emergence out of the natural sciences in the early twentieth century and its spilling over into the medical and social sciences at the end of that century. Following this historical and theoretical detour we shall turn directly to applying different concepts of complexity to the management of diabetes. Each chapter will take a particular complexity concept (complexity mapping, Stacey diagram, fitness landscape), provide a brief definition, explain how it is different from earlier orderly concepts and then explore how it can help, inform and improve existing diabetes management strategies and policies.

In no way will this be a complete or extensive review of all of the tools of complexity or their relevance to diabetes management. That is beyond the scope of this book. Rather it is designed to be an easily digestible 'taster' of what complexity thinking can provide. If you want more, there is a huge literature on complexity to explore, and short reading lists are provided at the end of each chapter. Hopefully, by the end of the book you will have seen enough connections between complexity and your own world for you to want to find out more.

This is just the beginning. It will be a long ride and we don't know exactly where it will lead, but it will be exciting and definitely better than putting on the blinkers of the orderly framework and complaining every time the diabetes rollercoaster won't go straight!

Reference

1 NICE Health Technology Appraisal on Patient Education; www.nice.org.uk/page.aspx?o=68326 (accessed June 2006).

Chapter 1

Diabetes and its treatment: yesterday and today

Diabetes . . . a melting down of the flesh and limbs into urine. . . . The course is a common one . . .; for the patients never stop making water. . . . The nature of the disease then is chronic, and it takes a long period to form, but the patient is short-lived if the constitution of the disease be completely established; for the melting is rapid, the death speedy.

(Aretaeus the Cappadocian, second century AD)[1]

The [diabetic] patient has a continual thirst, with some degree of fever; his mouth is dry, and he spits frequently a frothy spittle. The strength fails, the appetite decays, and the flesh wastes away till the patient is reduced to skin and bone.

(Dr William Buchan, *Domestic Medicine*, 1785)[2]

Diabetes mellitus is a condition in which the amount of glucose (sugar) in the blood is too high because the body cannot use it properly. Type 1 diabetes develops if the body is unable to produce any insulin. . . . Type 2 diabetes develops when the body can still make some insulin, but not enough, or when the insulin that is produced does not work properly (known as insulin resistance). . . . The main aim of treatment of both types of diabetes is to achieve blood glucose, blood pressure and cholesterol levels as near to normal as possible.

(Diabetes UK, 2006)[3]

Diabetes is not new and has been a serious plague on humanity throughout recorded history. It is a permanent and chronic condition. You either have it or you don't, and there is no such thing as mild diabetes. It invades individuals' lives both day and night without respite, and at the present time there is no known cure. Control is therefore the aim, but the experience of trying to control diabetes is like riding a 'rollercoaster' that never ends. This ride covers 'hypos' and 'hypers' associated with the lifestyle staples of diet and exercise, not to mention other normal life experiences such as illness, stress, hormonal changes and even temperature fluctuations. Alongside these are the effects of drug treatments – tablets and/or insulin injections. *Balance* is the key word. It acknowledges and captures the juggling act that self-management entails to achieve the balance of blood glucose control, alongside control of lipids (fats, including cholesterol) and blood pressure. This need for balance stems from a very simple fact – that the innate mechanisms for maintaining normal blood glucose levels within the body have gone awry. If uncontrolled, this can lead over time into cascading detrimental effects on organs within the body, most notably the eyes, kidneys, nervous system and heart.

In many ways the aim of balancing diabetes is no different to the multiple balances that everybody has to maintain in life in terms of what they eat and drink, and the amount of activity they maintain. What is different, however, is that with diabetes the balances are essential and more difficult to maintain. In essence, achieving 'balance' is similar to trying to drive on a busy road. The driver must stay within the road boundaries and follow certain rules to prevent accidents happening. It could be said that for people with diabetes, the road boundaries are tighter than for others, and this requires more 'rules', or at least good adherence to the 'rules.' Such discipline provides the challenges – mental, physical and social – of learning to self-manage or DIY the condition. Overcoming these challenges is not easy! As one patient wrote:[4]

> You come in, they say 'Oh, you've got diabetes . . .' and you are running round like your tail's been cut off thinking 'What am I going to do?'

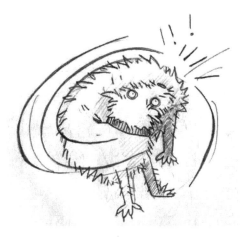

The demanding regime and its intimate relationship with day-to-day activities mean that the individual is much more responsible for, and in control of, the disease process. In essence, self-management is the 'cure', since it helps to prevent the very real risks of complications associated with the disease. The problem with learning how to balance this complex picture is that it takes more than just memorising when and what medicines to take and what foods to avoid. No one can live a life so regimented that diabetes could be perfectly controlled. So how can a patient or a carer with no biomedical background make informed decisions about the condition?

To answer this question we need to step back, cover a few basic points and take a brief look at the history of diabetes and its treatment.

Bad and good news

Fact 1

The onset of diabetes relies upon a combination of genetic and environmental 'triggers', such as inadequate nutrition or poor eating habits. In developing countries, starvation affects the intrauterine development of infants, which leads to the development of diabetes in later life. In the developed world, obesity, in particular central body fat (the 'apple shape') is strongly linked to insulin resistance. In the latter case, the body produces insulin, but is unable to use it properly. These two opposing dimensions – starvation and obesity – are the main reasons behind a frightening rise in diabetes worldwide.

Fact 2

Numerically, the disease is reaching epidemic proportions. A study that looked at all 191 World Health Organization (WHO) member states found that the prevalence of diabetes for all age groups worldwide was 2.8% in 2000 and estimated to be 4.4% in 2030. The total number of people with diabetes is projected to rise from 171 million in 2000 to 366 million in 2030. The study findings indicated that the 'diabetes epidemic' will continue even if levels of obesity remain constant. However, given the rising levels of obesity, it is likely that these figures are an underestimate of what the future will hold. Diabetes, it seems, is a global plague that can affect anyone – no one is impervious to the disease. It is a serious condition for the individual, and its rapidly increasing prevalence is a significant cause for concern. The most important factors contributing to this growing prevalence are ageing, urbanisation (predominantly in developing countries), sedentary lifestyle and increasing prevalence of obesity.[5]

Fact 3

These large numbers are obviously associated with high costs – in particular, hospital admissions to deal with the long-term complications of the condition. In many cases these complications could and should have been prevented. In the UK, for instance, close to £1 in every £10 is spent on treating diabetes and its complications in hospitals. Overall estimates of costs in the year 2000 amounted to 9% of National Health Service (NHS) costs – that is, £5,185,314,000. This is equivalent to:

- £99,717,567 a week
- £14,245,367 a day
- £593,560 an hour
- £9,893 a minute
- £165 a second.[6]

Fact 4

Despite a number of medical advances, patient self-management remains the cornerstone of diabetes treatment. Unfortunately, self-management is not only complicated and challenging, but can be very time consuming. A recent American study found that 'more than three hours a day would be required for an average type 2 diabetes patient to follow to the letter all the home-care tasks recommended.' They found that on average 96 minutes were needed for monitoring blood glucose, record keeping, medication management, foot care, problem solving and exercise, and a further 106 minutes per day were needed for meal planning, shopping and preparation.[7] Such findings highlight the personal effort and cost involved in successfully managing diabetes – a few pills or injections just won't do it.

Fact 5

There is some good news. Happily, the rates of complications have begun to decline in many parts of the world. This is due to several factors, including more sophisticated screening techniques such as the digital eye-screening cameras, innovative treatments such as the statin drugs – described as the new cholesterol-lowering 'antibiotic' – and improved specialist care due to adoption of international benchmarks aimed at improving disease management.[8] However, despite all of these advances, we still haven't found effective answers to controlling the rise in prevalence of the disease, its management and escalating costs. Why not? To answer this question, we need to explore what has gone on before.

Diabetes: the historical perspective

Diabetes mellitus has been around for a long time. In 1500 BC, early Egyptian healers noted that ants were attracted to the urine of people with a mysterious wasting disease from which children died very quickly and older people struggled with devastating complications. The 'Ebers Papyrus', an Egyptian document written in the late third century BC, first documented it as a condition 'without retention', and Apollonius of Memphis coined the word 'diabetes', meaning 'to go through', sometime around 250 BC. Other descriptions included that of Galen, a disciple of Hippocrates in the first century AD, who described it as 'diarrhoea of the urine' and the 'thirsty disease.' However, not until 1425 did the word 'diabetes' appear in an English book. By 1670, over 100 authors had written about it.[9,10]

During the seventeenth and eighteenth centuries, researchers began to explore the diagnosis of diabetes and the role of insulin. Thomas Willis in 1674 and later Matthew Dobson in 1776 identified the presence of sugar in the urine and thereby a means of diagnosing the disease. Willis proposed that the sugar appeared first in the blood and then later in the urine, and Dobson provided experimental evidence that confirmed this hypothesis. The descriptive word '*mellitus*' (Latin for 'honey'), was later added by Cullen in 1769 to separate it from *diabetes insipidus*, which refers to excess urination without sugar, a completely different disease. Other researchers of note include Claude Bernard in 1857, who identified the vital role of the liver in diabetes through the location of *glycogen*, the body's 'hidden' store of glucose. Paul Langerhans located what were subsequently called the *islets of Langerhans* in the pancreas as the body's production line for insulin. A number of people were involved in the isolation of insulin, '*iletin*' as it was originally called, and its role in lowering blood glucose in dogs from which the pancreas had been removed. They included the Romanian, Paulescu, and the better-known Canadians, Banting, Best, McLeod and Collip. Eli Lilly and Company started commercial production of insulin in America in 1923. In the 1930s, research by Himsworth clearly demonstrated the difference between type 1 and type 2 diabetes. In the 1950s, the first oral medications for type 2 diabetes were developed, and since that time a variety of convenient blood testing and diagnostic tools have been developed.

Looked at from this perspective, the diagnosis and understanding of diabetes are clearly a triumph for traditional scientific medicine. Knowledge and understanding have grown over time. More and better treatment options are available, and a vaccine for type 1 diabetes prevention is even being developed! Yet the disease refuses to go away. In fact, as we have seen, due to lifestyle choices (at least in the wealthy parts of the world) diabetes is now at epidemic levels. How can all of this increased knowledge not lead to better management and control of what is an escalating problem world-wide?

Fundamentally, as will be explained more thoroughly in the following chapters, diabetes is a complex condition that is intimately linked to the genetic disposition, body type, actions and lifestyle of the individual. Its onset and progression depend on a variety of interacting factors. Given this, matching 'cause' and 'cure' for diabetes becomes almost impossible.

Treating diabetes: from variety to order and back again

Unsurprisingly, in ancient and even comparatively recent times, the management of diabetes involved a wide array of treatments. In 1769, Buchan (author of *Domestic Medicine*,[2] such a popular book that it went through 100 editions) suggested that patients should wear flannel to help them to perspire, have regular 'gentle purges' of the bowels, drink alum in tea four times a day, and take moderate exercise. In 1866, George Harley MD of University College London outlined a very restricted diet for people with diabetes aimed at eliminating all sugars, by which he meant 'not only the avoidance of all sugars, and substances containing saccharine matter, but also of all kinds of food convertible during the process of digestion into sugar.'[11] Only green vegetable and animal products were allowed. Interestingly, at this time Harley noted that the key problem with maintaining the diet was stopping people from eating their favourite breads! One Italian diabetes specialist in the late nineteenth century, Catoni, had to keep his patients under lock and key in order to get them to follow their diets. In 1901, Dr John Morrisey wrote in the *Journal of the American Medical Association* that:

> So far as the treatment of diabetes is concerned, it is in a very chaotic condition. After using strontium [a bright silvery metal] and the other preparations provided by the genial manufacturer, I find that it is best to rely upon opium or one of its various preparations.[12]

Obviously, despite the recognition of the central importance of diet, a wide variety of other medicines and treatments – some useful, some neutral and some harmful – were explored.

However, with the discovery of insulin, its commercial availability in the 1920s and the advent of tablet treatments in the 1950s, medical experts became increasingly convinced that they could finally control the disease – provided, of course, that patients adhered to strict lifestyle instructions. Complications could be eliminated! In essence, like other traditional scientists of the time dealing with complex problems, the answer lay in simplifying and controlling as much of the process as possible. This approach is known as reductionism. So if doctors knew that the disease was interwoven with the habits of the patient and that they couldn't control the disease, they could at least control the patient!

This led to a number of strict dietary, insulin and exercise regimes that were often forced on passive patients. A quote from RD Lawrence (co-founder of Diabetes UK in 1934) on the 'red and black line diet' in 1932 provides a glimpse of the strict diet regimes that were popular at the time:

> Your doctor will prescribe a certain number of rations a day and tell you how many to take at different meals. One ration is one complete line, and consists of one black and one red portion. Any black portion can be added to any red portion to make one ration, but two black portions or two red portions must not be combined to make a ration. Thus equal numbers of blacks and reds must be taken together . . .[13]

The 'line diet' neatly affirmed the 'expert' knowledge of the doctor and the passive position of the patient who was supposed to follow the doctor's rules. Given this level of control, failure to comply was the patient's fault. Some patients puritanically revelled in the need for 'self-control.' HG Wells (of *War of the Worlds* fame, and co-founder of Diabetes UK in 1934 with RD Lawrence, who like him had diabetes) wrote:

> Our characters are strengthened by a perpetual self-control . . . for my own part I have certainly found diabetes an invigorating diathesis.[14]

As the century wore on, the line diet was replaced in the 1950s by the 'carbohydrate exchange system', a system that required a restricted carbohydrate (starch and sugar) 'prescription' so that the patient had to learn the carbohydrate content of foods to be able to balance insulin intake with food input.[15] This regime was equally controlling. However, by the 1980s even as blood glucose testing and the taking of insulin became easier, evidence was mounting to show that strict dietary regimes were unnecessary. In response, a more flexible 'healthy eating' plan was introduced in the 1990s, guided by the 'plate model':

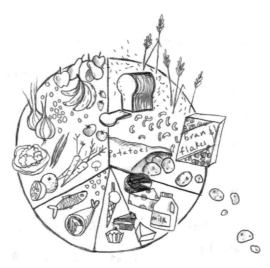

More recently, the fashionable Glycaemic Index – the GI Plan – has come into favour. This is a nutritional approach based on the ranking of foods according to their overall effect on blood glucose levels. Slowly absorbed foods have a low GI rating, and foods that are quickly absorbed have a high GI rating. Interestingly, the exchange system has now come back into fashion through education programmes such as 'Dose Adjustment For Normal Eating' (DAFNE), which encourage more flexible eating patterns alongside self-directed insulin doses.

What was slowly being learned by the medical profession was that despite their fundamental scientific training, it was not possible to solve a complex disease by simplifying the patient – because patients aren't simple! At a minimum, patients get hit by a vast array of normal life events that make constant rigid control of diabetes impossible. As one patient made clear:

> Everything can't be perfect all of the time, they do not know what's going on in your life that can upset things.[4]

Moreover, patients forget, make mistakes, resist, hide and dissemble in order to make their own world fit with the 'controlled' one of the medical expert. As a patient with type 1 diabetes reminiscing about dealing with medical visits as a child clarifies:

> Together with my parents, I quickly learnt how to play their 'game.' Hospital appointments required organisation: time to get the coloured pens out and concoct a diary of urine testing results that reflected variable but acceptable control; time to walk a few miles to the hospital so that the one-off blood glucose test (no long-term glycosylated haemoglobin tests then) was normal to low. The medical team were pleased with my 'success' and the status quo was maintained.

Today: focusing on balance rather than control

Today's situation is still about prolonging life but with an added twist – to maintain quality of life for people with diabetes *and* to work towards preventing onset of the disease, and its associated complications. This approach incorporates a complex array of activities that embraces not just treatment but also prevention, research, administration and, of course, education to support the key to diabetes control – patient self-management.

Self-management in real life remains both the essence of the treatment plan and the arena of patient expertise. It is a highly contextualised experience. As such, each individual has their own personal ideas about how to manage it, who to turn to for support, and which sources of information provide the most accessible routes to understanding. There are therefore a multitude of explanatory frameworks around self-management which are underpinned by a range of philosophies, alongside personal and professional ideas of how service users (patients and carers) and service providers (health professionals) should behave.

What this means is that professionals, patients and carers – all experts in their own right – need to move away from the traditional mechanistic way of viewing diabetes management:

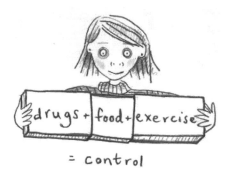

$= \text{control}$

Instead, they need to move towards one that recognises the 'random effects of life', and the key role of 'patient self-management.' Moreover, the 'equation' should realise that the end point is not some form of perfect control, but a continual adjusting balance of basic rules, patient learning and normal life changes and challenges:

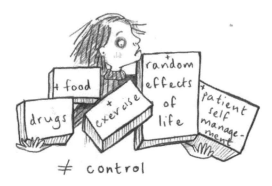

$\neq \text{control}$

Such an approach reflects the need for all involved in diabetes care – patients, carers and health professionals – to link cause and effect so that blood glucose control can be seen as a 'fit' between advice and patient compliance or, to give it its official name, patient 'concordance.' This term embraces the concept of patient empowerment, which is currently considered to be central to all healthcare activities. Empowerment is about sharing decision making – it is about working in partnership so that patients can make informed decisions about their health. It should therefore account for patients' self-perceived needs and their voluntary choices. This recognises that patients are both the producers of health and the customers of healthcare, and that patients, unlike health professionals, have expertise in 'living' with the disease. Although such a philosophy is not new in the field of diabetes, health professionals are still struggling with how to put it into practice.[16]

It is important to note that the multi-faceted nature of diabetes management has been around for some time. RD Lawrence noted in 1932 that:

> In the successful treatment of diabetics the patient, the nurse, the practitioner and the specialist are often partners working together to establish the patient's health. In the long run the most important part, the melody, is played by the patient, and the accompaniment may be almost unheard.[13]

This image of diabetes management as a partnership based on the interdependence of patients, carers and healthcare practitioners is now a part of mainstream thinking with regard to the future direction for diabetes care. However, with this view comes the need to develop a workable framework so that everyone can see the larger picture – one that brings all the actors and pathways together.

An international perspective

Without a doubt, diabetes is taken very seriously across the world. For example, in Europe, the St Vincent Declaration (SVD)[17] for the first time set international targets for the prevention of complications associated with diabetes. The SVD was an agreement of all European countries, under the auspices of the World Health Organization (WHO) and the International Diabetes Federation (IDF), to improve care for people with diabetes. The Declaration recognised the increasing incidence of diabetes on a global scale, and the associated rising economic costs of diabetes care, over and above its toll in terms of human suffering. It formulated a series of recommendations which embodied both general goals and specific targets for improvement in the health of those with diabetes. These guidelines became a real concept in the diabetes world, with 50 official national liaison people being appointed for the SVD Action Programme, alongside 15 working groups, and about 40 national diabetes action plans being formulated. In the UK, for instance, the government developed a Diabetes National Service Framework (NSF), which outlined 12 explicit standards for diabetes care and policies for execution, with working groups developing implementation plans for each standard.[18,19] In addition to these, there is a vast array of supportive materials available to both professionals and the public that can be easily accessed via the Internet. Of particular note is the UK digital National Electronic Library for Health (www.nelh.nhs.uk), launched in 2000, which provides access to the best current knowledge and know-how to support healthcare-related decisions.

However, despite all of these efforts, progress has been slow. In 2003, the IDF in Europe came to the conclusion that many of the agreed goals were either not reached or were ignored. A questionnaire on diabetes programmes in each country was distributed in December 2003, and the results showed that 'too many European countries are still discussing plans'[17] – obviously not doing enough, if anything. This lack of progress raises two questions.

- If so much attention and effort is being focused on diabetes, why is it still causing so many difficulties?
- Are we really doing anything different to what was being done before?

To answer the first question, one has to begin by recognising that the disease hasn't changed, but that people have. The disease is now recognised as being even more complex, with recognition of the intricate networks of variables that can interact to produce complications, necessitating even more lifestyle 'controls.' However, in most of the world, lifestyles have altered to such a degree that the disease has spread like wildfire. Fundamentally, this implies that no matter how many diabetes institutes, frameworks, agencies, standards, etc. governments decide to set up, these will only have a real impact if people begin to alter their basic lifestyles. In other words, addressing the scourge of diabetes means changing the attitudes of the general population towards a healthier lifestyle. This is a hugely complex policy problem that better diabetes treatments will do little if anything to alter.

Secondly, despite all of the evolving infrastructures, nothing fundamental has changed in our approach to diabetes. The prioritised areas have always been around, plus or minus a few others. The emphasis may therefore shift, and certainly the evidence base underpinning them has improved, but we are still on a moving escalator – one that must respond to crises at the same time as working on prevention and treatment under the limitations of a restricted NHS budget. The endless list of agencies and treatments embodies this. It is obvious that something else is needed. This 'something' needs to provide people 'at the coalface' – patients, carers and practitioners – with a way of comprehending what is happening to them. The information is out there. The question is, can it be put together in a new way that really makes sense.

Here we come to our key point. We believe that complexity science offers a way out of the current impasse. It will not cure diabetes. It will not reduce the complexity of patient self-management. It will not eliminate tensions between professionals, patients and carers over diabetes management. However, it can shift the framework for understanding the condition and the relationship between the key actors by stressing that the complexity of diabetes and its management is really very normal. In fact, dealing with complex events and processes makes up the majority of our lives. Our physical, biological and social worlds are filled with them. All of us are experts in complexity.

What happened from the eighteenth century onwards was that a clockwork, mechanical and orderly vision of the world founded by Newton set the framework of modern science and medicine. As we shall see in the next chapter, this mechanical framework viewed disease as a mechanical process that could be controlled with the proper 'inputs' and actions. Diabetes could be managed if we only listened to the medical experts and controlled ourselves enough. From a complexity perspective, since life (and disease) is basically complex, more control does not automatically lead to a better, healthier life. Balance, learning and adjusting are what life is really all about. Recent changes in diabetes care, as a mark of progress, all point to a growing acceptance of the complexities of diabetes and a more or less unconscious awareness of complexity thinking. What is amazing is that despite the growing recognition of the complexity of diabetes and its treatment, many medical experts and patients still seem determined to find ways of returning to the belief that some sort of rigid control will provide a final answer. We do not believe in this false hope. In fact, as Catoni demonstrated by imprisoning his patients to make sure that they followed his diet, rigid order is often just a cage.

The expert in all of us

The diabetes experience is similar and different for every patient. There is something to learn in every case. Coping strategies are particularly unique. A simple example of this lesson of complexity can be found in the narrative of an adult reminiscing about dealing with diabetes as a child when first diagnosed.

Looking back . . . a child's perspective

Catherine was diagnosed with type 1 diabetes at the age of 8. She has lived with diabetes for nearly 40 years. She has two children, works full time and lives a very full life.

> When in the first throes of diabetes, I remember that it wasn't easy to make sense of the new language, particularly as a young child. Terms like insulin, pancreas, islets of Langerhans, hypoglycaemia, hyperglycaemia, ketoacidosis, blood glucose, dietitians, lipids and carbohydrates do not make for easy listening. Alongside this, the impact of a lifetime diagnosis of a disease that is associated with potential 'nasty' complications and a series of rituals including injections and urine (now blood) testing is not easy to accept. In hindsight, the words 'stunned, scared, sorrowful' were very appropriate to my newly acquired label. Having strange, obtrusive feelings that could not be articulated within the confines of an 8-year-old vocabulary led to the development of new medical terminology. Feeling 'shaky' meant having a 'hypo', feeling 'sugary' was associated with 'hyper' status, 'not fair' meant I was grieving and in need of loving support. I also assigned 'real-life' status to injections (boilable glass syringes and metal reusable needles at this time), 'telling them off' if they hurt and threatening them with the bin if they did it again! Urine testing was seen as a ritual to be endured and referred to only as 'testing', with no use of an embarrassing toilet word. It was a time of great confusion. It felt like I had entered a 'story' world, a story because it was happening to someone else – it didn't feel real.

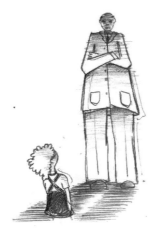

References

1 Aretaeus the Cappadocian, cited by Morrisey J in *History of Diabetes*; www-unix.oit.umass.edu/~abhu000/diabetes/index.html (accessed June 2006).
2 Buchan W. *Domestic Medicine, or a Treatise on the Prevention and Cure of Diseases by Regimen and Simple Medicines.* Exeter: JB Williams; 1785.

3 Diabetes UK. *Understanding Diabetes: what is diabetes?* www.diabetes.org.uk/diabetes/under.htm (accessed June 2006).

4 Cooper H. *Capturing the impact of patient education for people with type 2 diabetes.* PhD Thesis. Liverpool: University of Liverpool; 2001.

5 Wild S, Roglic G, Green A *et al.* Global prevalence of diabetes. Estimates for the year 2000 and projections for 2030. *Diabetes Care.* 2004; **27:** 1047–53.

6 Currie CJ, Kraus D, Morgan CL *et al.* NHS acute sector expenditure for diabetes: the present, future, and excess in-patient cost of care. *Diabet Med.* 1997; **14:** 686-92.

7 Shubrook JH, Schwartz FL. American Diabetes Association, 66th Scientific Session; http://scientificsessions.diabetes.org/index.cfm?fuseaction=Custom.Content&MenuID=1000 (accessed June 2006).

8 Krans HMJ, Porta M, Keen H. Diabetes care and research in Europe. The St Vincent Declaration Action Programme. *G Ital Diabetologia.* 1992; **12(suppl 2):** 32–6.

9 Sanders LJ. From Thebes to Toronto and the twenty-first century: an incredible journey. *Diabetes Spectrum.* 2002; **15:** 56–60.

10 MccCracken J, Hoel D. From ants to analogues. *Postgrad Med Online.* 1997; **101;** www.postgradmed.com/focus_on/diabetes.htm (accessed June 2006).

11 Harley G. Cited in Morrisey J. *History of Diabetes;* www-unix.oit.umass.edu/~abhu000/diabetes/index.html (accessed June 2006).

12 Morrisey J. *History of Diabetes;* www-unix.oit.umass.edu/~abhu000/diabetes/index.html (accessed June 2006).

13 Lawrence RD. *The Diabetic ABC. A practical book for patients and nurses.* London: HK Lewis and Company Ltd; 1932.

14 Grady W. Wells laid foundation. *Balance.* 2005; **207:** 44–6.

15 Rogers IH. *The Complete Cookery Book for Diabetics.* London: Whitefriars Press Ltd; 1956.

16 Cooper H, Booth K, Gill G. Patients' perspectives on diabetes health care education. *Health Educ Res.* 2003; **18:** 191–206.

17 International Diabetes Federation. *St Vincent Declaration. Re-awakening the Saint Vincent movement;* www.idf.org/home/index.cfm?node=839 (accessed June 2006).

18 Department of Health. *National Service Framework for Diabetes: standards.* London: The Stationery Office; 2001.

19 Department of Health. *National Service Framework for Diabetes: delivery strategy.* London: The Stationery Office; 2003.

Chapter 2

What is complexity?

I think the next century will be the century of complexity.
Stephen Hawking (eminent physicist cited on www.comdig.org)

She blinded me with science. She hit me with technology.
Thomas Dolby (from 'She blinded me with science' a pop chart hit in 1983)

These two quotes nicely capture the problem of talking about complexity. On the one hand, it has been around for some time, is firmly established throughout the natural sciences and is even seen as a future dominant paradigm for the sciences. On the other hand, like all sciences, it often wallows in its own language, focuses on questions and concerns that do not easily relate to common human experiences, and is easily ignored and parodied by popular culture. This chapter focuses on bridging this divide. Complexity has a fascinating history that even a pop star can understand (though to be fair to Thomas Dolby, he was one of the most technically advanced stars of the 1980s).

So how do we begin? We all know what complexity means – sort of complicated only messier. The *Oxford English Dictionary* identifies complexity as a derivative of 'complex', coming from the Latin root *complexus*, and defines it as 'consisting of many different and connected parts . . . hard to understand, complicated.' However, complexity science is much more than this common definition. To understand complexity science and its relevance to medicine in general and diabetes in particular, we must take a slight detour through a few hundred years of intellectual history.

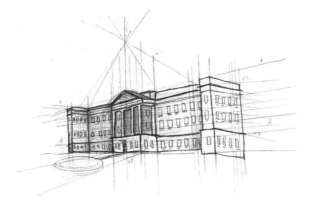

The vision of order

The seventeenth- and eighteenth-century Enlightenment was an astounding time for Europe. Relatively stagnant and intellectually repressed during the so-called Dark

Ages, the intellectual energies released by the Renaissance came to fruition in the Enlightenment. During this time, Europe was reborn and became the centre of an intellectual, technical and economic transformation. Science was liberated from centuries of control by religious stipulations and blind trust in ancient philosophies. The Frenchman René Descartes (1596–1650) and, slightly later, the Englishman Sir Isaac Newton (1642–1727) set the scene. Descartes advocated the power of human reason and its inherent rationality, while Newton unearthed a wondrous collection of fundamental laws of nature. A flood of other discoveries in diverse fields such as magnetism, electricity, astronomy and chemistry soon followed, injecting a heightened sense of confidence in the power of human reason to tackle any situation. Later, the eighteenth-century French scientist Pierre Simon de Laplace (1749–1827) pushed the orderly nature of the Newtonian framework to its logical conclusion by arguing that 'if at one time, we knew the positions and motion of all the particles in the universe, then we could calculate their behaviour at any other time, in the past or future.'[1] From this, Laplace implied that human beings could know not only the present, but also the past and the future.

The irony of these thinkers of natural and human order is that their lives were anything but orderly. Descartes hated to get out of bed and would often work in it all day. He later died of pneumonia when forced to get up at 5am by the Queen of Sweden. Newton produced most of his intellectual work during a five-year period in his twenties. Much of the rest of his life was spent trying to turn lead into gold, fighting with other intellectuals and promoting a small Christian sect. Laplace struggled to keep his head on his shoulders during the French Revolution.

The subsequent phenomenal success of the Industrial Revolution in the eighteenth and nineteenth centuries, which was based on this new vision of order, created a high degree of confidence in the power of human reason to tackle any physical situation. By the late nineteenth and early twentieth century many scientists believed that few surprises remained to be discovered. For the American Nobel Laureate, Albert Michelson (1852–1931), 'the future truths of physical science are to be looked for in the sixth place of decimals.'[2] Implying that there was a finite amount of knowledge, humanity had already found most of the fundamental bits, and there really weren't many more important things to learn about the universe. Science had lost its romantic appeal. It was like being a clockmaker and only being able to play with the small gears.

To simplify, this vision of an orderly universe was founded on four golden rules.

- **Order:** given causes lead to known effects at all times and places. (Dropping a ball from my hand will lead to the same effect – hitting the floor – no matter where I am on Earth or what time I do it.)
- **Reductionism:** the behaviour of a system can be understood, clockwork fashion, by observing the behaviour of its parts. (There are no hidden secrets to a mechanical clock. The parts move and the hands tell the time. Parts can be separated.)
- **Predictability:** once global behaviour is defined, the future course of events can be predicted. (If the clock works perfectly, assuming no breakdowns, we can know where the hands will be at midnight, noon, 8am, and so on.)
- **Determinism:** processes flow along orderly and predictable paths that have clear beginnings and rational ends. (The hands of the clock start when we add energy to them by plugging in the clock, winding it up, etc. The hands only go around the

dial – they don't make erratic movements or jump off the dial – and they stop when the energy supply runs out.)

From these golden rules a simple picture of reality emerged as shown in Figure 2.1.

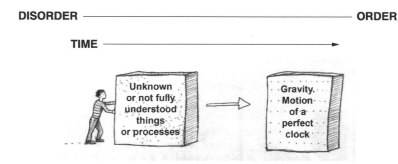

Figure 2.1: Phenomena in the vision of order.

Given the golden rules and the picture of reality, several expectations emerged.

- Over time, as human knowledge increases, we shall realise that the world is more and more orderly.
- With greater knowledge/order, humans can increasingly predict and control more and more phenomena.
- There is an end point to the universe and hence to knowledge.
- Science (and knowledge) is orderly. It is hierarchical (some bits are more important than others) and can be divided into academic disciplines (e.g. natural sciences vs. social science and arts) or medical specialisms (e.g. paediatrics vs. surgery vs. geriatrics).

This last point is particularly important, since it implies that scientific knowledge is fundamentally different from and superior to common or everyday knowledge, that knowledge can be divided into separate domains (called departments in universities or specialties in medicine) and that there is a hierarchy in the sciences as well. As the Nobel prize-winning physicist Ernst Rutherford famously said, 'All science is either physics or stamp collecting.' Now the big question for you is how all of this relates to diabetes.

The natural sciences spill over into the social and medical sciences

Not surprisingly, success in these areas had a profound effect on attitudes in all sectors of human activity, spreading well beyond the disciplines covered by the original discoveries. The human and social sciences were no exception. Surrounded by the technological marvels of the Industrial Revolution, it did not take much of an intellectual leap to apply the lessons of the physical sciences to the social world. Academics in all the major fields of social science welcomed the new age of certainty and predictability with open arms. Economics, politics and sociology all became 'sciences', desperate to duplicate the success of the natural sciences. Moreover, this desire was institutionalised through the development of modern departmentalised universities.

In the fields of biology and human anatomy, the Italian physiologist Borelli (1608–1679) argued that:

> as the scientific recognition of all these things is founded on geometry, it will be correct that God applied geometry by creating animal organisms, and that we need geometry for understanding them.[3]

From this perspective, the body became just another type of mechanism – much more complicated than clocks, but fundamentally no different. The trick to under-standing and controlling the body (correcting its mistakes) was to reduce it to its component parts and find tools for understanding and measuring its 'motions.' Whereas in the seventeenth century medical diagnosis was based heavily on listening to the patient's interpretation of his or her condition, by the eighteenth and nineteenth centuries a growing array of technological innovations (e.g. the micro-scope, stethoscope, blood-pressure monitors, X-ray machine, etc.) 'encouraged a physical separation of the doctor from his patient.'[4] With the growing technological advances of the late nineteenth and early twentieth centuries, medical laboratories and centralised hospitals began to proliferate, as well as the routine use of a wide array of medical testing procedures. Testing not only became a way of objectively evaluating the patient and protecting the doctor from charges of malpractice, but it even allowed doctors to feel that they were 'using the same rigorous methods as did the scientist who pursued truth in his laboratory.'[5]

Linked to this 'scientification' of medicine was the growth of specialisation. Specialisation was the logical outcome of the growing detailed knowledge of the human body combined with the belief that it was fundamentally a mechanical clock that could be separated into its key components. Large-scale medical institutions would bring together all of these specialisms into a 'one-stop' body shop! Eventually, with the growth of computers, more and easier testing and greater knowledge, disease could be eliminated as it was in the science fiction TV programmes and films of the 1960s and 1970s – *Star Trek, Logan's Run* and *Star Wars* to name just a few well-known (and maybe even embarrassing) examples. All it would take would be a wave of the doctor's computer-enhanced wand.

Science and society don't stand still

Certainty and predictability for all – the hallmarks of an orderly frame of mind – were too good to last. Cracks had existed for some time, and even Isaac Newton and Christiaan Huygens in the seventeenth century couldn't agree on something as fundamental as the nature of light (whether it is a particle or a wave). These difficulties bubbled under the surface of acceptable scientific discourse and the expanding university arenas. They were often seen as unimportant phenomena that would be resolved by the next wave of emerging fundamental laws. However, by the early twentieth century they could no longer be ignored. Henri Poincaré (1854–1912), the supreme physicist of his age, was one of the first to voice disquiet about some contemporary scientific beliefs. Later, the theory of relativity of Einstein (1879–1955), the quantum measurement problem of Erwin Schrödinger (1887–1961) and the uncertainty principle of Werner Heisenberg (1901–1976) all played a decisive role in pushing conventional wisdom beyond the Newtonian limits that had enclosed it centuries before. These scientists, all Nobel laureates, set in motion a process that eventually transformed attitudes in many other disciplines.

The new discoveries revealed that not all phenomena were orderly, reducible, predictable and/or determined. What this meant was that even at the most fundamental level, some phenomena do conform to the classical framework, while others do not. With this revelation, the boundaries of the classical paradigm were cast asunder. Gravity continued to function and linear mechanics continued to work, but they could no longer claim to be universally applicable to all physical phenomena. They had to exist alongside phenomena and theories that were essentially *probabilistic* – that is, providing probable solutions to problems rather than certainties. Causes and effects are not directly linked – the whole is not simply the sum of the parts. Taking the system apart does not reveal much about its overall behaviour, and the related processes do not steer the systems to inevitable and distinct ends.

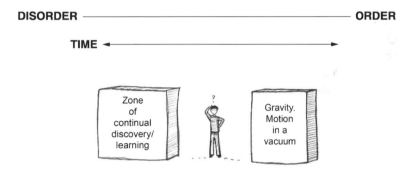

Figure 2.2: Phenomena in the paradigms of disorder and order.

Given these complex phenomena and their non-adherence to the golden rules of order, new expectations were necessary for this expanding paradigm.

- Over time, human knowledge may increase, but phenomena will not necessarily shift from the disorderly to the orderly.
- Knowledge does not always equal order. Greater knowledge may mean the increasing recognition of the limits of order/knowledge.
- Greater knowledge does not necessarily impart greater prediction and control. Greater knowledge may indicate increasing limitations to prediction and control.
- There is no universal structure/end point to phenomena/knowledge.

It is important to note that the shift in scientific analysis from utter certainty to considerations of probability was not accepted lightly. High levels of specialisation meant that even scholars involved in the same discipline were not immediately aware of discoveries being made by their colleagues. Moreover, the language of science itself became almost unintelligible beyond a select circle of specialists, and their intriguing speculations were not at first thought to be of everyday concern. Nevertheless, uncertainty was eventually recognised as an inevitable feature of some situations. In effect, the envelope of orderly science was expanded to add complex phenomena, also known as *complex systems*, to those that were already in place.

Complexity in the physical world

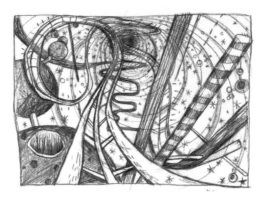

Once the door was open to probability and uncertainty, a new wave of scientists began studying phenomena that had previously been ignored or considered secondary or uninteresting – Rutherford's 'stamp-collecting' activities. Weather patterns and fluid dynamics were just two of the areas that saw the growing acceptance of non-linear complex phenomena and systems. For example, one of the earliest people to conceptualise and model a complex system was the American meteorologist, Edward Lorenz. In 1961, he developed a computer program for modelling weather systems. However, to his dismay, due to a slight discrepancy in his initial program, the program produced wildly divergent patterns. How was this possible? From an orderly linear framework, small differences in initial conditions should lead to only small differences in outcomes. Yet in Lorenz's program, small discrepancies experienced feedback and reinforced themselves in chaotic ways, producing radically divergent outcomes. Lorenz called this phenomenon, whereby small changes in initial conditions lead to radically divergent outcomes in the same system, the 'butterfly effect', arguing that given the appropriate circumstances a butterfly flapping its wings in China could eventually lead to a tornado in the USA. Small causes did not always lead to small effects. Order was not certain. Chaos/complexity was an integral part of physical phenomena.

One of the most famous and simple examples of this type of fluid-based complex system is the Lorenzian waterwheel. This is a wheel that pivots around a centre point and has hanging buckets at the wheel's rim. There are holes in the bottom of each bucket, and water is poured in from the top. If the flow of water is too low, the bucket will not fill, friction will not be overcome and the wheel will not move. If the flow is increased, the buckets will fill and the wheel will spin in one direction. However, if the flow is increased to a certain point, the buckets will not have time to empty on their upward journey. This will cause the spin to slow down and even reverse at uneven intervals. Thus even a simple mechanical system can exhibit chaotic non-linear behaviour. Riding the diabetes rollercoaster is very similar to the motion of Lorenz's waterwheel – small changes (e.g. in diet) can have big effects that can turn a 'hypo' into a 'hyper', or a life-building challenge into a personal catastrophe.

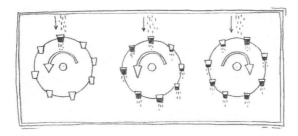

It is important to note that these systems are not necessarily complicated or random. Orderly systems are found at or near equilibrium. A ball bearing inside a bowl is a classic example – it quickly settles at the bottom and that is that. However, these systems can be very complicated. A jet engine is a wonderfully complicated piece of orderly machinery which creates highly predictable physical outcomes that millions of pilots and passengers successfully depend upon every year. Complex systems may be very simple but never settle into a final stable point – equilibrium. A basic example of this is the height of sand piles on a table. Consider a continual stream of sand that is pouring on to a common table (say 1 metre in diameter). The sand will generally form a pile that is around half a metre high (depending on the sand, the conditions, etc.). However, the height of the pile will continuously vary as small avalanches occur due to the continually added sand pouring on top. After a very short time, you can roughly predict the height of the pile in the future, give or take 20 centimetres. However, even if you watch it for a very long time – for years – you will still find it very difficult to improve on your predictions, as each new grain of sand combines with the pile in a unique way. This is the simplest form of complex system.

The range of physical phenomena can be visualised as shown in Figure 2.3.

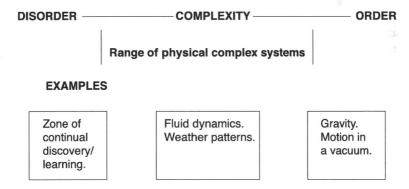

Figure 2.3: The range of physical phenomena in a complexity paradigm.

Box 2.1 Golden rules for physical systems in a complexity framework

- **Partial order:** phenomena can exhibit both orderly and chaotic behaviours.
- **Reductionism and holism:** some phenomena are reducible to their parts (e.g. mechanical clocks), while others are not (e.g. water flows).
- **Predictability and uncertainty:** phenomena can be partially modelled, predicted and controlled.

- **Probablistic:** there are general boundaries to most phenomena, but within these boundaries exact outcomes are uncertain. The best experts can do is to say what is likely to occur, or probable.

Complex systems in the living world

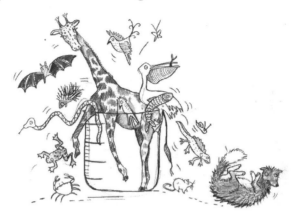

By the latter half of the twentieth century, with complexity already deeply penetrating the physical sciences, biologists, geneticists, environmentalists and physiologists also began to consider their respective disciplines within the context of complexity. Analysts in these fields set out to investigate the properties of systems, including human beings, comprised of a large number of internal parts that interact locally in what looks like a state of anarchy that somehow manages to engender self-organised, stable and sustainable global order. These systems are not only complex but also adaptive, and display *emergent properties* or *emergence* (i.e. the creation of a new structure or process).

Unlike non-living physical phenomena, the ability of biological or living complex systems to adapt and evolve creates a whole new range of complex outcomes. The Lorenzian waterwheel discussed above does display unpredictable movement, but it could run for ever and it will never change into a different waterwheel. Living biological systems have the ability to fundamentally alter over time, from single cell to multi-cellular organisms, from dinosaurs to birds, and from primates to humans. Just give them enough time and who knows what will evolve!

A simple example of a biological complex system would be the evolution of a species or the interaction of a given plant or animal in a particular ecosystem. A fish in a small pond will evolve and interact with the various food sources (small plants and animals) in the pond to create a stable complex system (e.g. a stable total number of fish). However, if a change is introduced to the system (e.g. a new competitor or food source), the fish may adapt and alter the nature of the system in totally unforeseen ways. Over time, new emergent properties may evolve in the system and/or in the fish itself. The fish may develop powerful eyes for seeing the bottom of the pond, giving it a comparative advantage over other fish. A larger example is that of the concept of *Gaia* developed by James Lovelock. For Lovelock, the Earth was not a ball of rock with a layer of life on the surface, but a huge organism that combined physical and biological properties in very complex patterns and demonstrated fascinating emergent behaviour – from the large-scale interaction of plant and animal life to the responses to occasional massive extraterrestrial influence (large meteorites, not alien invasions!).

Due to the emergent nature of biological systems, the level of complexity can be significantly higher than that of non-living physical phenomena and systems. Therefore, on our simple scale of complexity, biological complexity is placed on the more disorderly side of the scale relative to physical complexity.

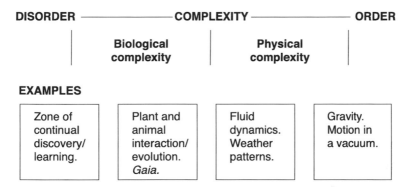

Figure 2.4: The range of physical and biological phenomena.

Box 2.2 Golden rules for biotic systems in a complexity paradigm

- **Partial order:** phenomena can exhibit both orderly and chaotic behaviours.
- **Reductionism and holism:** some phenomena are reducible, whereas others are not.
- **Predictability and uncertainty:** phenomena can be partially modelled, predicted and controlled.
- **Probabilistic:** there are general boundaries to most phenomena, but within these boundaries exact outcomes are uncertain.
- **Emergence:** these systems exhibit elements of adaptation and emergence. New plants and animals emerge out of the old.

Complexity in the human world

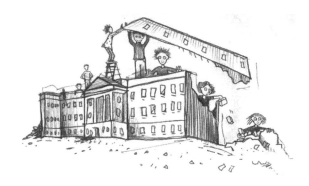

Despite the dominance of the orderly framework, there continued to be a huge variety of potent critics of the mechanical view of nature and society and of the limits of human rationality. In the late eighteenth century, Immanuel Kant (1724–1804), the German scientist and philosopher, argued that an organism 'cannot only be a machine, because a machine has only moving force; but an organism has an organising force . . . which cannot be explained by mechanical motion alone.'[6] In the late nineteenth and early twentieth century, Sigmund Freud (1865–1939) and Max Weber (1864–1920) challenged the belief in human rational capabilities and the degree to which humans can understand and control their environment and society. In the 1960s, the Nobel prize-winning economist FA Hayek argued that 'in the field of complex phenomena the term "law" as well as the concepts of cause and effect are not applicable.'[7] Consequently, from the 1970s onwards as social scientists continually failed to capture the 'laws' of society and economic interaction, and were continually frustrated by their inability to do so, they began to significantly question the Newtonian framework.

The fields of medicine and health were no exceptions in moving away from the more orderly and mechanical framework. As early as 1876, Theodor Billroth was worried that:

> The object of our modern endeavour is to make the physician's skill . . . independent of the talent of the individual and may be reduced to an absolute science. All knowledge and skill are to be determined and controlled by means of the laws of arithmetic and logic in order to make everything absolute and permanent. . . . I doubt if this good will ever be reached, at least in the art of healing.[8]

Not long afterwards, other doctors actively opposed the growing diagnostic testing and specialisation of medicine for overshadowing the importance of personal knowledge of the patient. For example, in 1905 Richard Cabot established the first social service department in American medicine at the Massachusetts General Hospital to train social workers and doctors to explore how patients' personal and social situations affected their health. Of particular relevance is Cabot's conclusion regarding a patient with diabetes:

It was useless to hand her out a diet-list without finding out whether she can get at her boarding-house any such diet as we recommend. It turns out that she cannot, that there is no boarding-house for diabetics, and that she had no money to spend on specially selected diets. Shall we simply pass to the next case and let the woman's disease run on to its fatal termination unimpeded? The physician in charge has no time to investigate her case. . . . He needs the help of social workers to make his treatment effective.[9]

Similarly, in 1919 a leading medical practitioner, Sir James Mackenzie, was arguing that 'the conception of specialism dominant today is a wrong one . . . instead of enlightening, it tends to darken in a cloud of detail.'[10] More recently, experts have increasingly recognised that specialisation produces its own problems of fragmentation of care. This growing concern over the increasing fragmentation of care is neatly captured by the words of one frustrated patient with multiple complications, dealing with different specialists, who said to them 'Do none of you [specialists] talk to each other?'[11] Finally, others rejected the fundamental notion of specialisation which assumes that the body is no more than the sum of its various parts and that greater specialisation represents medical progress. As medical historians have pointed out, specialisms and specialisation have risen and fallen over time. According to one historian, the society with the greatest degree of specialisation was that of the Ancient Egyptians![12]

But how do human beings fit into the complexity paradigm? Obviously they are part of the complex web of their physical and biological surroundings, but what makes them distinct from this environment? Their most fundamental difference is consciousness – the ability to ask 'Who am I?', 'How did I get here?' and 'What does life mean?' This ability to be self-aware, to understand aspects of the world around them, to be aware of their history and to evolve interpretations of themselves and their surroundings makes human beings fundamentally different from all other life forms and physical phenomena. However, this advanced ability to interpret themselves and the world around them does not produce unified or orderly interpretations. The uniqueness of individual human experience combined with multitudinous possibilities of collective human interaction and the evolutionary nature of human society produces an incredible variety of interpretations or human stories. A simple glance at the competing cultures that make up our world, let alone the diverse opinions that can be found in our own neighbourhood, clearly demonstrates the power of human diversity. Therefore conscious interpretive outcomes (norms, values, historical interpretation) must be positioned on the more disorderly side of our complexity scale. This does not imply that there are no universal norms, values or interpretations. For example, a prohibition against murder is a common societal trait. However, the definition of murder, the mitigating circumstances that could surround it and the punishment for the act all vary widely over time and between different societies and cultures. The position of conscious phenomena is outlined in Figure 2.5.

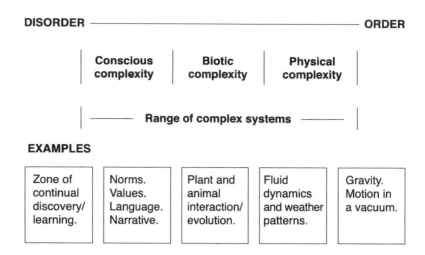

Figure 2.5: The range of physical, biological and conscious phenomena.

Box 2.3 Golden rules of conscious systems in a complexity paradigm

- **Partial order:** phenomena can exhibit both orderly and chaotic behaviours.
- **Reductionism and holism:** some phenomena are reducible, whereas others are not.
- **Predictability and uncertainty:** phenomena can be partially modelled, predicted and controlled.
- **Probablistic:** there are general boundaries to most phenomena, but within these boundaries exact outcomes are uncertain.
- **Emergence:** they exhibit elements of adaptation and emergence.
- **Interpretation:** the actors in the system can be aware of themselves, the system and their history, and may strive to interpret and direct themselves and the system. *You* make a difference just by being *you*!

How does this relate to everyday human events?

The next step is to explore how this relates to everyday human life. Using Figure 2.5 as a template, we can produce an overview of the range of complexity dynamics of human phenomena. The key point to recognise is that there are both orderly and disorderly dynamics and that they are not hierarchically organised. A given human outcome – a decision to have coffee at breakfast or to bomb a particular village – could be based on orderly, complex and disorderly dynamics, with all being equally essential to the final outcome.

Beginning with orderly dynamics, the most fundamental and universalistic elements of human complexity are basic physiological functioning, in particular life and death. These physical boundaries and requirements – carbon-based life forms requiring air, water and food in order to survive and reproduce – are the most orderly aspects of human existence. Deprived of these fundamentals, a human will die. What could be more orderly?

Moving into the range of complex systems, examples of mechanistic complexity in human systems would involve situations where individuals are forced to act in a mechanistic fashion. Traffic dynamics (choosing one road or another), crowd dynamics (choosing one exit or another) and electoral outcomes (choosing one candidate or another) are all examples of mechanical complex systems. These systems are relatively simple and stable patterns will emerge. However, this is no guarantee that these patterns (traffic jams, crowd delays, landslide elections) will be continuously stable, nor is it possible to perfectly recreate the exact conditions of these events at a later time. The golden rules of physical complex systems apply.

Examples of biological complex systems in the human world can easily be seen in the organisational dynamics of economic and social institutions. As demonstrated by the huge growth in management and complexity literature, a business is a complex system that interacts with a larger complex environment (the market) that is very similar to the earlier model of a fish in a pond. General patterns emerge and the business is able to adapt to changes in its environment, but exact predictions and explanations of how a change in the environment will affect the business, or the best strategies for the business to survive in the altered environment, are impossible to know in advance.

An added layer of complexity in the human condition is its faculty of consciousness. Human beings create signs, symbols, myths, narratives and discourse in order to understand, control and exchange information about their surroundings. This ability adds another layer of complexity to the human condition that is distinctive from the natural world. Examples of this conscious complexity include the creation of language, norms and values and discourse, and can be taken from virtually any type of human verbal interaction. A seemingly simple student–teacher relationship can be layered in historically, culturally and personally specific aspects that would be impossible to recreate in a different time and place.

Lastly, like the natural world, disorderly human phenomena are nearly impossible to explain using examples, since they are without a pattern and would have to be completely random. These could range from the influence of random events to the chaotic nature of dreams and the unconscious, random effects of certain disorders on the complex functioning of the brain, and the phenomena of luck. In essence, this is the ultimate area of individual experience that is constantly in the process of discovery and learning. (*See* Figure 2.6.)

How can all of these dynamics be combined to explain everyday human phenomena? Let us begin with a simple daily event – going to a shop to get a cup of coffee and something to eat. You have a basic human need for water and nutrition that is very orderly and highly predictable, particularly for those with diabetes. This is combined in the case of the coffee with the desire for a mildly addictive stimulant and a snack to maintain normal blood glucose levels. As you leave home to walk to the coffee shop, you immediately encounter crowd dynamics that may speed or impede your journey to the shops. When you reach your favourite coffee shop, you see that a new coffee shop has opened on the opposite corner of the street, competing for your business. These shops are engaged in the complex biological process of competition. In a process of conscious complexity, you are enticed to enter the new shop by its pleasant name, 'Vic's Coffee Shop', which reminds you of a childhood friend. As you enter the shop a woman is leaving with a cup of coffee. You open the door for her and say 'good morning.' As she turns to thank you a fly lands randomly on your face and you

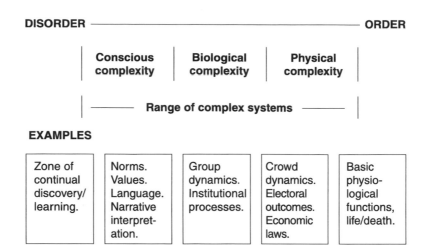

Figure 2.6: The range of complexity systems in human phenomena.

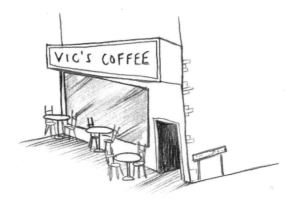

immediately flinch, accidentally hitting the woman so that she spills her coffee all over your clothes. You return home, embarrassed by the stains and worried that you need food quickly in order to avoid a hypo. You have a quick snack and change your clothes, but given all of the 'mess' you forget to have a cup of coffee! The point of detailing this pursuit of coffee is to demonstrate the remarkable orderly, complex and disorderly processes that are the foundation of most commonplace, everyday events in human life.

The amazing and even entertaining thing about a complexity framework is that you can apply it to virtually any aspect of human life and trace out the orderly, complex and disorderly bits. What this shows is that complexity is really the science of common

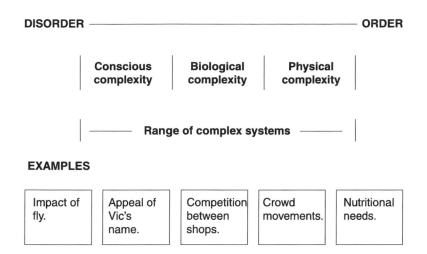

Figure 2.7: The range of complexity in everyday life.

sense, and that we are all experts in complexity. We deal with it on a constant basis, from the physical demands of our bodies to the social demands of our partners, families and work colleagues. The strange thing is that despite all of this complexity, many individuals, societies and scientific frameworks in particular seem desperate to find some sort of certainty or final order in their lives, systems or structures. In many ways, it is the pursuit of this 'final order' that leads to much worse individual and social outcomes than the original uncertainty and complexity.

Now this may be very interesting, but the obvious question still remains. How does all of this relate to diabetes and the triangular relationship between the patient, the carer and the health professional? To answer this question requires a new chapter.

References

1 McEvoy JP, Zarate O. *Introducing Quantum Theory.* London: Icon Books; 2001. p. 159.
2 Horgan J. *The End of Science: facing the limits of knowledge in the twilight of the scientific age.* New York: Broadway Books; 1996. p. 19.
3 Mainzer K. *Thinking in Complexity: the computational dynamics of matter, mind and mankind.* 4th ed. Berlin: Springer; 2004. p. 96.
4 Reiser SJ. *Medicine and the Reign of Technology.* Cambridge: Cambridge University Press; 1978. p. 90.
5 Reiser SJ. *Medicine and the Reign of Technology.* Cambridge: Cambridge University Press; 1978. p. 162.
6 Mainzer K. *Thinking in Complexity: the computational dynamics of matter, mind and mankind.* 4th ed. Berlin: Springer; 2004. p. 97.
7 Hayek FA. *Studies in Philosophy, Politics and Economics.* Chicago: University of Chicago Press; 1967. p. 42.
8 Galdston I. *Social and Historical Foundations of Modern Medicine.* New York: Brunner/Mazel Publishers; 1981. p. 105.
9 Reiser SJ. *Medicine and the Reign of Technology.* Cambridge: Cambridge University Press; 1978. p. 178.

10 Galdston I. *Social and Historical Foundations of Modern Medicine*. New York: Brunner/Mazel Publishers; 1981. p. 86.

11 Carlise C, Cooper H. Do none of you talk to each other? The challenges facing the implementation of interprofessional education. *Med Teacher.* 2004; **26**: 545–52.

12 Galdston I. *Social and Historical Foundations of Modern Medicine*. New York: Brunner/Mazel Publishers; 1981. p. 87.

Further reading on complexity in general

The following is an easy book for beginners.

Sardar Z, Abrams I. *Introducing Chaos*. London: Icon Books; 2001.

The following are all advanced books, but well written.

Briggs J, Peat FD. *Turbulent Mirror: an illustrated guide to chaos theory and the science of wholeness.* New York: Harper and Row; 1989.

Byrne D. *Complexity Theory and the Social Sciences*. London: Routledge; 1998.

Casti J. *Complexification: explaining a paradoxical world through the science of surprise.* London: Abacus; 1994.

Coveney P, Highfield R. *Frontiers of Complexity: the search for order in a chaotic world.* London: Faber and Faber; 1995.

Gell-Mann M. *The Quark and the Jaguar*. London: Little Brown; 1994.

Gleick J. *Chaos*. London: Sphere; 1988.

Goodwin B. *How the Leopard Changed its Spots*. London: Phoenix; 1997.

Holland J. *Hidden Order: how adaptation builds complexity*. Cambridge, MA: Helix Books; 1995.

Kauffman S. *At Home in the Universe*. London: Viking; 1995.

Lewin R. *Complexity: life at the edge of chaos*. Chicago: University of Chicago Press; 1992.

Nicolis G, Prigogine I. *Exploring Complexity*. New York: Freeman; 1989.

Prigogine I. *The End of Certainty: time, chaos, and the new laws of nature.* New York: Free Press; 1997.

Waldrop M. *Complexity: the emerging science at the edge of order and chaos.* New York: Simon and Schuster; 1992.

Further reading on complexity and health

Fraser SW, Greenhalgh T. Complexity science: coping with complexity: educating for capability. *BMJ.* 2001; **323**: 799–803.

Goldberger AL. Non-linear dynamics for clinicians: chaos theory, fractals, and complexity at the bedside. *Lancet.* 1996; **347**: 1312–14.

Goldberger AL, Rigney DR, West BJ. Chaos and fractals in human physiology. *Sci Am.* **262**: 42–9.

Goodwin JS. Chaos and the limits of modern medicine. *JAMA.* 1997; **278**: 1399–400.

Holt T, editor. *Complexity for Clinicians*. Oxford: Radcliffe Publishing; 2004.

Kernick D, editor. *Complexity and Healthcare Organization: a view from the street.* Oxford: Radcliffe Publishing; 2004.

Lindberg C, Herzog A, Merry M *et al.* Life at the edge of chaos – health care applications of complexity science. *Physician Executive.* 1998; **January/February issue:** 6–20.

Matlow AG, Wright JG, Zimmerman B *et al.* How can the principles of complexity science be applied to improve the coordination of care for complex pediatric patients? *Qual Safety Health Care.* 2006; **15**: 85–8.

Plesk PE, Greenhalgh T. The challenge of complexity in health care. *BMJ.* 2001; **323**: 625–8.

Plesk PE, Wilson T. Complexity science: complexity, leadership, and management in healthcare organisations. *BMJ.* 2001; **323**: 746–9.

Steinberg D. *Complexity in Healthcare and the Language of Consultation: exploring the other side of medicine.* Oxford: Radcliffe Publishing; 2005.

Sweeney K. *Complexity and Primary Care: understanding its value*. Oxford: Radcliffe Publishing; 2006.

Sweeney K. Griffiths F, editors. *Complexity and Healthcare: an introduction*. Oxford: Radcliffe Medical Press; 2002.

Wilson T, Holt T, Greenhalgh T. Complexity science: complexity and clinical care. *BMJ*. 2001; **323**: 685–8.

Chapter 3

Learning how to use 'complexity mapping'

Where's the beef?
(TV actress Clare Peller in 1984 TV advertisement
for an American hamburger restaurant chain)

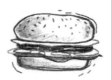

In the 1980s, a hamburger restaurant chain in the USA launched a TV advertising campaign with the theme '*Where's the beef?*' The advertisement's tactics were to take an elderly female actress and have her portray herself as the embodiment of a friendly but firm grandmother. She would politely listen to the outrageous claims about the size of the hamburgers, the variety of ingredients, and so on, of competing hamburger chains and then calmly but firmly ask the question '*Where's the beef?*' Having dealt with complexity thinking for several years, we are constantly being asked, in not exactly these words, '*Where's the beef?*' The remaining chapters of this book are all about responding to this question.

We can begin with the concept of 'complexity mapping.' Fundamentally, all it involves is taking the basic figures that were developed in the previous chapter and applying them to diabetes, the patient, carer and health professional, and the relationship between all of them. Using complexity mapping one can begin to explore the amazingly orderly, complex and disorderly interrelationships between the condition, the patient, their family and friends and healthcare professionals, and how these can be used to gain greater understanding of the range and 'balancing process' of the diabetes experience.

Health and the health system from an orderly perspective

Let us begin by turning to Figure 3.1 and making a quick comparison of what an orderly interpretation of health would look like in relation to a complexity interpretation.

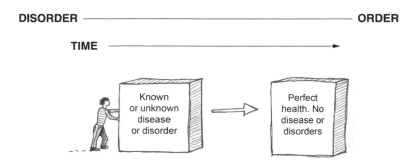

Figure 3.1: Health in an orderly perspective.

Given this perspective, our golden rules would be as follows.

- **Causality:** cause leads to effect. Eliminate disease and/or disorder, and health will improve.
- **Reductionism:** the parts of the system can be separated. Divide and isolate individual diseases and/or disorders, cure them, and health will improve.
- **Predictability:** outcomes can be known. A given pill or treatment will cure the disorder/disease and health will improve.
- **Determinism:** the path from illness to health is known. A given set of treatments, actions, etc. will cure the patient step by step, and improve health.

Now if we assume that health is fundamentally order, then we must make our health system fundamentally orderly as well. What would this look like?

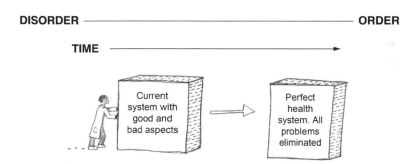

Figure 3.2: The health system in an orderly perspective.

The golden rules can be summarised as follows.

- **Causality:** increase the number and accuracy of government health targets in the health system and societal health outcomes will improve.
- **Reductionism:** government health targets can be separated and addressed individually.
- **Predictability:** if we put more money and effort into health it will automatically improve.
- **Determinism:** we know the exact steps necessary to improve the health of society in the long run.

Obviously, as discussed in Chapter 2, if these rules are true then we should have similar expectations.

- Over time, as human knowledge increases, more diseases/disorders will be eliminated, targets will eradicate health system problems, and general health will improve.
- With greater knowledge, humans, through their health system, can increasingly predict and control disease and disorders.
- Eventually there will come a time when all diseases and disorders will be eliminated by an orderly health system, and health will be perfect.
- Increased medical hierarchy and specialisation overseen by benign and rational government targets indicate growing control over health.
- **Extra point**: the role of the public and the patient in this perspective is passive. Experts have the knowledge. The best that the public and the patient can do is to 'do as they are told.'

Undoubtedly this is an extreme position. You would struggle to find a health professional or policy actor in the Department of Health who would say that everything is perfect. On the other hand, many would say that this vision of order is the underlying goal. For many policy actors, the key strategies are to isolate and study the problem, apply a target and evaluate the results. If the results are good, the problem is solved. If they are bad, a new target is tried, and so on, until the problem is solved. Health professionals often get locked into this logic as well – just take out the word 'target' and insert 'pill', 'treatment', etc. Remember that in many situations where the system, condition or disease is primarily orderly, these tactics and methods work reasonably well and have given society many of its major health breakthroughs. Think about vaccinations and antibiotics.

Health and the health system from a complexity perspective

But what if, as we have seen in the preceding chapters, health is not orderly? What would it look like then? To save a little time and space we shall jump directly into the full complexity perspective discussed in Figure 2.5 in the last chapter.

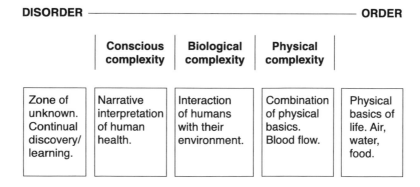

Figure 3.3: Health in a complexity perspective.

From this perspective, what would our various boxes mean? For example, moving from right to left, the most orderly aspects of human health are its physical basics. Remove air from humans and we die in minutes, remove water and we die in days, remove food and we die in weeks. How we combine these physical basics as individuals and as a society is a good example of physical complexity. The blood flowing through the human body makes innumerable complex movements going down one blood vessel or another, flowing from one organ or another. Likewise, the supply and flow of blood from blood banks to hospitals demonstrates a similar dynamic. Biological complexity is easy because it is so obvious. We are constantly interacting with an enormous variety of viruses, bacteria and animals, as well as other humans. Life is interaction. Similarly, conscious complexity is also clear. Health has meaning and what we mean by 'health' changes with place and time. The 'healthy-looking' six-pack of the modern male model, enhanced by exercise, contrasts markedly with the vision of a healthy 'stout' man of Victorian times. Lastly, there is always the element of the unknown in health – a new virus (think about bird flu), disease (think about MRSA) or fashion (think about new recreational drugs). It can all change in totally unpredictable ways.

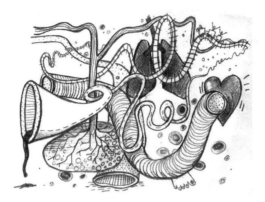

Given our complexity framework, what do its golden rules look like?

- **Partial causality:** phenomena can exhibit both orderly and chaotic behaviours. (Air, water and food still matter, but so do the multitudinous ways in which we combine them.)
- **Reductionism and holism:** some phenomena are reducible whereas others are not. (Flu viruses have a clear negative impact on some individuals, but how do they affect whole populations?)
- **Predictability and uncertainty:** phenomena can be partially modelled, predicted and controlled. (The fact that some diseases spread is clear, but exactly how they will spread is much less predictable – just like the weather.)
- **Probabilistic:** there are general boundaries to most phenomena, but within these boundaries exact outcomes are uncertain. (The general progression of a given disease has certain common boundaries, but how it will affect a given patient or population within those boundaries is less well known.)
- **Emergence:** they exhibit elements of adaptation and emergence. (Just like humans, viruses, bacteria and other living things change over time.)
- **Interpretation:** the actors in the system can be aware of themselves, the system and

their history, and may strive to interpret and direct themselves and the system. (We make a difference to the system just by being us.)

From here we can take a quick look at how a complexity perspective would view the existing health system.

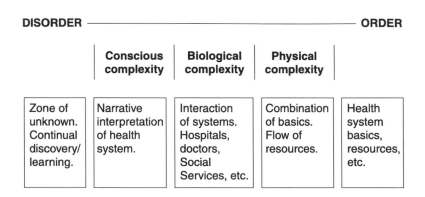

Figure 3.4: The health system in a complexity perspective.

In this case, moving again from right to left, the most orderly aspect of the health system is its basic resources. Does it have staffing, drugs and money? If so, how many or how much? These basics will set the boundaries of the system. Next, how are these resources combined and allowed to flow throughout the system? Further along, how do the main structures within the system interact, compete and evolve with each other? Do hospitals or community care services dominate? Do family doctors or hospital consultants benefit from changes in the system? Clearly, conscious complexity captures the social and political nature of the health system. Should it be free for all, privately or publicly owned, or insurance based? Do we have confidence in it? Do we like it? Lastly, and most unpredictably, what will the system look like in 10, 20 or 50 years' time? Remember that the British NHS is only in its fifth decade. Likewise, the American health system has been radically transformed in the period since the Second World War.

What do our golden rules for the health system look like from a complexity perspective?

- **Partial causality:** basic resources/targets matter – financial resources – but the amounts are always uncertain.
- **Reductionism and holism:** at best there are degrees of separation between aspects of the system (departments, specialisms, etc.).
- **Predictability and uncertainty:** fundamental changes do matter, but so may small ones. (Think of a change of habit with regard to washing hands leading to the spread of MRSA 'superbugs' in hospitals.)
- **Probablistic:** unknown long-term impact of all major changes to the system.
- **Emergence:** policy change creates new health system strategies, which create new policies, and so on.
- **Interpretation:** public opinion shapes health and the health system.

Now if we accept the complexity perspective, our expectations of and our role in health and the health system become very different.

- Health is a continual process. Knowledge may increase, but health, the health system and diseases/disorders will continue to change. Focus on creating an adaptive healthcare system rather than the final perfect one.
- Greater knowledge may or may not increase disease/disorder prediction and control. Learning how to cope with continual change and uncertainty is just as important.
- Health and the health system will never be perfect. The best health and health system are adaptive, flexible and learning entities.
- Increased medical hierarchy and specialisation and intrusive government targets do not indicate growing control over health. They have risen and fallen over time and may strip adaptability, flexibility and learning from the health system.
- **Extra point**: the role of the public and the patient in the complexity perspective is an active one. *You play a key role in generating the system and your own health.*

The last point is particularly important, and one of the most difficult to grasp fully. How can you be so important to a system and to your own health? Well, not only do you pay for the system and influence it in a variety of active and passive ways, but also the decisions that you make in your daily life generally far overshadow the occasional advice you receive from health professionals. Moreover, as the complexity perspective shows, experts with extensive knowledge are generally good at understanding and directing the orderly parts of health and the health system. However, as one moves to the more complex side of the scale, it is the public and the patient that should have a growing voice.

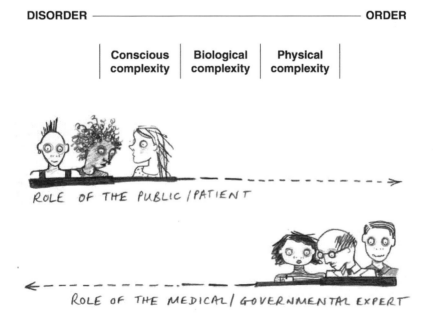

Figure 3.5: Decision making in a complexity perspective.

From health to diabetes: making the most of complexity mapping

Like the jump that complexity thinking is making from the natural to the social sciences, it isn't much of a leap from a complexity perspective on health and the health system to one on diabetes. Let us start by looking at how the orderly perspective views diabetes, the patient, the carer and the health professional.

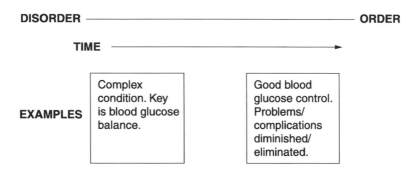

Figure 3.6: Diabetes in an orderly perspective.

The golden rules can be summarised as follows.

- **Causality:** managed diet, activity levels and insulin usage automatically lead to good blood glucose control – *more management equals greater control.*
- **Reductionism:** different aspects of diabetes management can be separated and addressed individually (e.g. diet, exercise, drug treatment).
- **Predictability:** more management, leading to greater control, will improve health.
- **Determinism:** more management, leading to greater control, will improve health and keep it that way in the long term.

Once again, given this perspective and these golden rules, what expectations should one have for diabetes and its treatment?

- Over time, more knowledge about diabetes will be generated by health experts through research.
- With greater knowledge, predictability, management and control over blood glucose levels will increase.
- Eventually, blood glucose control will be virtually perfect and diabetes will be effectively managed.
- To hasten this development, medical specialisation, research and government targets for diabetes eradication should increase.

Given these expectations, what are the roles of the various actors involved with diabetes. Clearly, the patient's role is passive. How can they possibly accumulate all of the knowledge necessary to understand this complicated condition? Their fundamental role is to provide accurate information to the health practitioner and to do as they are told. The patient's family and carers play a similar informational and extra enforcement role. They are to provide information if the patient is unable to (because he or she is too young or too old), and to ensure that the patient follows the medical instructions. Health practitioners play a mixed role of God and enforcer. If they are the high-level experts – diabetes specialists – they determine the exact dosages, procedures and actions to be taken. The responsibility and pressure are immense. Other actors – doctors and nurses – must follow this advice to the letter. Fundamentally, they are the key enforcers in the health system using whatever combination of inducements is necessary to get the patient to comply with the treatment.

An excellent example of this type of thinking can be found in a recent book on diabetes that told a story about a wise old professor giving a lecture on the importance of 'patient compliance.'

> One of the tough old internal medicine professors asked his class, 'What is the biggest problem in diabetes?' Of course, there are many problems in diabetes. After two students answered incorrectly, my friend raised his hand and sheepishly said, 'Patient compliance?'

> The professor was amazed and delighted my friend had answered this rather tricky question. Puzzled, the professor said, 'Wait a second. Did I have your brother in this class some years ago?'

> 'No, sir,' replied the student. Still, the professor was surprised this young student could get the answer right. When pressed, my friend finally admitted his father had been a student under the old professor and had passed down the lesson. My friend received an 'A' in the class.[1]

The obvious implication is that getting patients to do as they are told is not only the key problem for diabetes, but has been so for generations!

Admittedly, this is an extreme position. Patients and carers are rarely so passive. Diabetes experts would laugh if you suggested that they were 'gods.' And what reasonable doctor or nurse would say that their basic job in relation to diabetes patients is the same as that of a school matron presiding over an unruly group of students? Nevertheless, despite occasional protests, the orderly perspective pervades the health system.

It is even more pervasive in the treatment and care of diabetes, because the latter is so complex and unpredictable. This may seem nonsensical at first. Shouldn't such a complex condition demand a complex response? Not if you are an actor in an orderly system! Imagine the poor medical expert in this system. He or she is expected to produce perfect advice for every distinctive patient. It isn't possible. The only way out is to admit that the system is wrong or to find some way to blame people underneath you, including the patients. Doctors, nurses and other healthcare professionals are caught in the middle, trying to help patients as best they can, but also struggling to stay within the rules set by the experts. Lastly, there are the patients and the carers. They want to believe that if they just do as they are told, all will be well and they will return to some sort of normality, like before. Unfortunately, their lives are rarely so simple, and learning how to manage the disease requires more than just 'doing as you are told.'

What does diabetes look like from a complexity perspective?

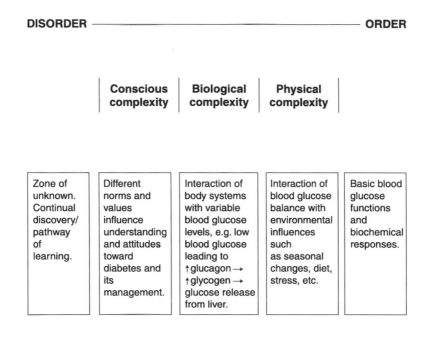

Figure 3.7: Diabetes in a complexity perspective.

As seen above, the most orderly aspects of diabetes are its fundamental chemical processes. For example, for people without diabetes, insulin released from the islets of Langerhans in the pancreas performs the balancing function of maintaining blood glucose levels in the body – so-called homeostasis. Take away the islet cells in the pancreas and we die. The body is in a continual state of biological complexity, with different systems and organs interacting with each other (witness the effect of low blood glucose levels) and responding to new external stimuli such as variations in temperature following seasonal changes. The malfunctioning of the pancreas for people with diabetes complicates this complex biological equilibrium by failing to balance the blood glucose levels, leaving the individual to manage this difficult task. The conscious side of diabetes is obviously not only the unique way in which every person faces their condition, but also their personal norms that influence disease self-management. For example, individuals with diabetes in societies that disapprove of alcohol consumption do not face the same social discomfort as those in societies that do consume large amounts of alcohol. Or an athlete who is used to monitoring their daily food intake and activity levels may be better able to deal with the balancing aspects of diabetes than a more sedentary person. Lastly, the zone of uncertainty is obviously the unique way in which each person who has diabetes approaches self-management of their condition, and ultimately how they come to terms with having the disease.

What do our golden rules for diabetes look like through a complexity perspective?

- **Partial causality:** basic management matters, but more management does not always lead to greater control.
- **Reductionism and holism:** at best, degrees of separation between different aspects of diabetes management (diet, temperature, activity, mood, etc.) all interact to some degree to influence blood glucose levels.
- **Predictability and uncertainty:** fundamental strategies do matter (e.g. following a healthy diet), but so may minor ones (e.g. changing an injection site).
- **Probablistic:** the long-term impact of most major strategies for dealing with diabetes is unknown.
- **Emergence:** life changes (e.g. puberty, pregnancy or menopause) require different management strategies.
- **Interpretation:** individual and public opinion shapes diabetes and its management.

Now if we accept the complexity perspective, our conceptions and strategies for dealing with diabetes take a different turn.

- Diabetes management is a continual process. Public and individual knowledge of the condition may increase, but the condition, its management and people with diabetes themselves will continue to change. The focus should be on creating adaptive and evolving responses to diabetes rather than final perfect ones (e.g. 'needs assessment' for deciding what education is required for individual patients).
- Greater knowledge of diabetes may or may not increase disease/disorder prediction and control. Learning how to cope with its continual change and uncertainty is just as important.
- Diabetes management will never be perfect. Even if diabetes was to be 'cured', obese individuals who tend to get type 2 diabetes would probably experience other health problems. The best responses to diabetes are adaptive, flexible and learning ones for patients and professionals alike.
- Increased medical specialisation (more diabetes experts) and intrusive government targets (more government management) do not guarantee improved control over diabetes. If they merely impose a more orderly vision of diabetes, they may inadvertently block patient adaptability and learning and actually worsen individual and overall diabetes management.
- Extra point: the role of the public and the patient in diabetes management from a complexity perspective is active. *You play a key role in managing diabetes and your own health.*

All of this can be surprisingly simplistic yet at the same time overwhelming.

For many health practitioners and people who have lived with diabetes for a long time, all of this is blatantly obvious and just plain old 'common sense.' They have been dealing with this type of complexity for years. They know all about it. So their thoughts take us back to the beginning: '*Where's the beef?*' For these actors, the 'beef' in complexity is the knowledge that they are not alone, that they are not fighting the one and only scientific structure, that their gut feeling and constant struggles against 'orderly' actors and the opinions of the latter are just as 'scientific' as gravity. It just took the medical profession and social sciences a little time to catch up with them!

For newly trained health professionals and newly diagnosed patients all of this complexity may be frighteningly overwhelming. Insecurity and a fear of failure may trouble the new health professional, while fear, anxiety and loss can distress the newly diagnosed individual. The key lessons to remember are as follows.

You are not alone. Diabetes is a major health challenge. There are millions of people with the condition! All of them are going through a similar but individually unique process. It is scary and disturbing, but it is up to you to work through the difficulties and realise that no one's health is ever fully stable. We never stop changing, adapting and adjusting until we are dead (an orderly state if ever there was one).

You have done this before. No, of course you haven't had diabetes before. However, you have dealt with hundreds, thousands, maybe millions of new complex and adaptive situations from the very beginning of your life. Dealing with siblings, learning to ride a bicycle, starting a new school, going through puberty, getting married, having your own children, getting older and, yes, even dying are complex learning processes. Fundamentally, *you* are a complexity expert already!

Blindly following the rules won't solve your problems. Fundamentally, dealing with diabetes is no different from learning a new sport. First, you have got to learn the rules, watch others play, talk to other players and listen to your coach, and then you just have to have a go. Later, as your confidence and experience grow, you can safely explore different tactics and strategies. This doesn't mean that they all work, just that you know how to deal with them when things go wrong. Most importantly, as any sportsperson will tell you, the rules are merely guidelines. Stretching, bending and pushing them is what creates a good player. Diabetes is no different. The game is how to manage your diabetes and make the most out of your life. There are some basic rules, but where you go from these is basically up to you!

Diabetes can be a lifetime companion, not a lifelong enemy. As discussed above, human life is a continual process of balancing physical, biological and social systems and needs. Diabetes complicates that balance, but does not fundamentally alter it. Life is always full of joyous and frightening complexity. The key point is what you do as you work your way through it.

Thought experiment: mapping your own complexity

This chapter has focused on exploring the use of the 'complexity map' (the row of boxes) for moving readers' minds away from their traditional orderly 'map.' Nevertheless, as any educational expert will tell you, the only way in which people really learn is if they integrate the lesson into their own lives. To do this we strongly encourage you to complete the following mapping exercise. Use the row of five boxes and put yourself in it. You can put in a long-term perspective or the current events of today. Either way, the basic structure remains the same. Hopefully, it will help you to separate the different aspects of complexity and realise that once you break it down, you really are a complexity expert. Moreover, you may find it useful to imagine what a carer, family member or the family doctor or nurse would be in a complexity perspective. Compare the results and see what you learn. There is no right answer. Just going through the process is what really counts.

Case study

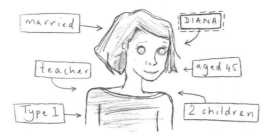

Imagine Diana, a 45-year-old teacher who is married with two children and has had type 1 diabetes for 28 years. She is visiting her family doctor for a regular check-up, but is worried that her blood glucose levels have been a little hit and miss lately. The basic attributes of her life are stable (she is married, etc.). However, she is wondering whether she should alter her injections, diet or exercise, or all three, in order to improve things. On the other hand, she is also concerned that her son seems to be increasingly embarrassed about her having diabetes. Could this be affecting her? More importantly, she has just begun a new job after spending many years at home caring for her children, and although she is enjoying it, she is finding it stressful at times. Is this the root of the problem? And if it is, what can she do about it anyway? (*See* Figure 3.8.)

Henry is Diane's doctor. He has known her for 6 years, from when he joined the surgery, and has felt that she dealt with her diabetes fairly well. He has several patients with type 1 diabetes and has read up on some of the latest research, but is more at home with type 2 patients. During his meeting with Diane he checks and confirms that her basic diet, insulin usage and exercise regime are OK. He listens carefully to her concerns about her son and the new job. Both are obviously causing her some degree of stress, and he knows that this can affect her diabetes. However, how this occurs and what to do about it are both very unclear to Henry. He doesn't have children and he rarely deals with teenagers. In the end, he listens and tries to be encouraging by saying that she appears to be doing OK. He offers some guidance on stress management strategies. He really doesn't know what else to say or do, and is reluctant to alter her insulin dosage, given his lack of experience. In her own way, Diane knows all of this, but she is reassured nonetheless.

William is Diane's 14-year-old son. He loves sport and is just discovering that teenage girls are very interesting. Previously he was never very worried about his mother's diabetes. She seemed to deal with it well and it never seemed to interfere with his life. However, he did hate it when he saw her injecting herself. Lately, Will had been attracted to a beautiful girl, Carrie, in his art class, and had been struggling to find some excuse to meet with her. Will's mother is an amateur painter. When Will mentioned this to Carrie, she said that she would love to meet her and see her work. It was the perfect opportunity. But Will kept putting it off. Was it that introducing Carrie to his mother was so bad, or was he embarrassed about his mother's diabetes? What if Carrie saw his mother injecting or, even worse, having a hypo?

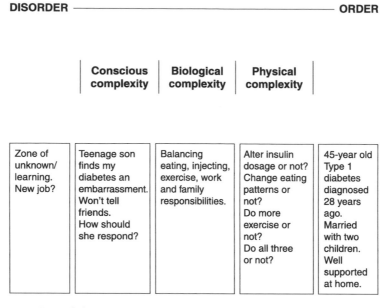

DISORDER ——————————————————————— **ORDER**

Conscious complexity	Biological complexity	Physical complexity

Zone of unknown/ learning. New job?	Teenage son finds my diabetes an embarrassment. Won't tell friends. How should she respond?	Balancing eating, injecting, exercise, work and family responsibilities.	Alter insulin dosage or not? Change eating patterns or not? Do more exercise or not? Do all three or not?	45-year old Type 1 diabetes diagnosed 28 years ago. Married with two children. Well supported at home.

Figure 3.8: Imaginary diabetic in a complexity perspective.

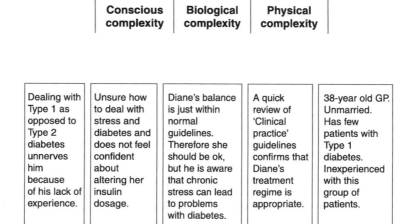

DISORDER ——————————————————————— **ORDER**

Conscious complexity	Biological complexity	Physical complexity

Dealing with Type 1 as opposed to Type 2 diabetes unnerves him because of his lack of experience.	Unsure how to deal with stress and diabetes and does not feel confident about altering her insulin dosage.	Diane's balance is just within normal guidelines. Therefore she should be ok, but he is aware that chronic stress can lead to problems with diabetes.	A quick review of 'Clinical practice' guidelines confirms that Diane's treatment regime is appropriate.	38-year old GP. Unmarried. Has few patients with Type 1 diabetes. Inexperienced with this group of patients.

Figure 3.9: Imaginary health professional in a complexity perspective.

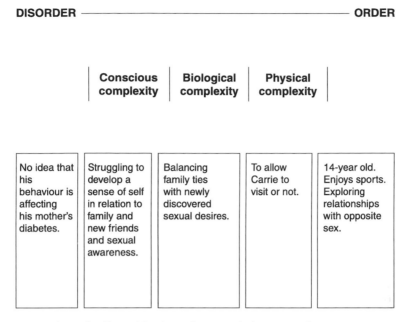

Figure 3.10: Imaginary family member/carer in a complexity perspective.

Reference

1 Juliano J. *When Diabetes Complicates Your Life: controlling diabetes and related complications.* Minneapolis, MN: Chronimed Publishing; 1998; p. 78.

Chapter 4

Learning to play the right 'mind games': moving from anxiety to balance

We're playing the mind games together
Pushing the barriers, planting seeds
Playing the mind guerilla
Chanting the mantra peace on earth
We all been playing those mind games forever
Some kinda druid dudes lifting the veil
Doin the mind guerilla
Some call it magic the search for the grail.

John Lennon[1]

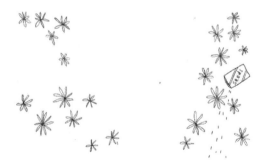

Ok, it is a bit 1970s, but John Lennon's song – *Mind Games* – encapsulates the many questions that 'living' generates, and the constant search for finite answers. 'Mind games' are a common attribute of all human beings as we try to sort things out and resolve problems. Try reflecting on conversations you have had with yourself and with others in recent weeks. You may recall many questions that have been raised – a close friend looking at how she can juggle work and home life, a colleague looking for the best way to lose weight, a neighbour trying to find how to reduce the amount of litter in your street, and alongside these your own concerns about how you can care effectively for your ageing parents, and what to do with your teenage children next weekend.

Individually none of these strikes you as extraordinary. You know that with time they will settle down and may even be resolved on their own or with help from others. Such experiences are commonplace. As Kutchins and Kirk[2] wrote, 'You recognise that these routine problems provide the bumpy texture of human life.'

However, for people living with diabetes, the 'bumpy texture of human life' is plural rather than singular. Their everyday experiences occur alongside self-management of a chronic disease. They live within a psychological predicament. Being diagnosed with the disease imposes a lifelong burden, yet diabetes is a 'hidden' disease – no one can see it – and expectations are that the individual will continue to lead a 'normal' life.

Some people living with diabetes may, quite rightly, argue about such concepts of 'normality.' Is it normal to watch what you eat everyday? Is it normal to inject insulin up to four times a day or to take tablets regularly? Is it normal to self-monitor blood glucose levels? Is it normal to routinely watch for hypos and hypers? Is it normal to live under the threat of potential nasty complications?

This chapter is about exploring these issues – the 'mind games' that diabetes plays. It is focused on exploring these games from both a traditional perspective and a complexity perspective, so that you can decide which best answers your questions.

A couple of facts

To begin this journey, let us look at some published facts about, and a central problem with, the psychology of diabetes.

Fact 1: What you think and feel about diabetes is important

Diabetes provides an additional risk factor for developing psychological problems. The prevalence of mental health problems in people with diabetes exceeds that found in the general population. Negative attitudes, coping difficulties, eating disorders, depression, anxiety and other disorders frequently complicate healthcare and are often missed.[3,4] Poor psychological functioning causes suffering, can seriously interfere with daily diabetes self-management,[5] and is associated with poor medical outcomes and high costs.[6,7]

Fact 2: This is now officially recognised

For example, in the UK the importance of addressing the psychological needs of patients and their families has been acknowledged by the government, albeit indirectly, through the underpinning philosophy of 'patient empowerment.' Rosie Winterton, Minister of State for Health Services in the UK, made a speech in 2005 in which she said:

> Empowering people with diabetes is at the core of the Diabetes National Service Framework (NSF). Let people have personal control and experience the best possible quality of life. As one diabetes patient has been quoted in the past as saying, 'I want to live with diabetes, not suffer from it.' That is the goal of the Diabetes NSF.[8]

Key to achieving the goal of empowerment is patient education and inter-disciplinary teamwork – drawing on the combined knowledge and skills of a multi-disciplinary team.

However

Fact 3: The majority of studies of the psychology of diabetes have segmented the emotional realities of coping with diabetes

Strange but true, most psychological work has divided the emotional effects into separate compartments mirroring the typical specialisation of healthcare systems. For example, studies have focused on efforts to identify a diabetes personality and a compliant personality,[9] alongside evaluations of grief reactions to diabetes and the concept of chronic sorrow – a response to ongoing loss.[10] There has also been interest in patients' health beliefs,[11] their individual coping mechanisms[12] and their personal models of illness,[13] to name but a few – and, of course, the effects of all of these on blood glucose control based on the rationale that psychological factors impact indirectly on control through behaviour. This diversity is reflected in the many questionnaires that claim to measure psychological 'bits and pieces' such as quality of life, well-being, treatment satisfaction, fear of hypoglycaemia, knowledge and cognitive function, attitudes and beliefs, psychological adjustment, perceived control, behaviour, social–environmental factors, barriers to self-care, and self-management.[14] Unsurprisingly, as they lack an underlying framework that can unite these diverse aspects, all of these studies have resulted in a lack of agreement about the relative importance of the psychological impact of diabetes.

Fact 4: Psychological care is far from adequate

A large cross-sectional research study of people with diabetes and healthcare providers in 13 countries in Asia, Australia, Europe and North America in 2005 showed that diabetes-related worries were common among patients, but few (only 10%) reported receiving any psychological treatment. From the health providers' perspectives, they found that although they recognised patients' worries, they reported not having the resources to manage them. The authors therefore concluded that psychosocial problems are common among people with diabetes worldwide, that addressing these problems may improve diabetes outcomes, but that providers often lack critical resources for doing so, particularly skill, time and adequate referral sources.[15]

Here we see the central problem or contradiction with current diabetes care. The real burden of coping with the emotional challenges of diabetes primarily rests with the patient and their family. Essentially, then, it is DIY psychological care – make your own way through the 'mind games.' From anybody's perspective this might not look too good coming from health services that are trying to work on the principles of promoting health and preventing disease.

So we are left with a fragmented view that tells a story of diabetes-related 'mind games' failing to be tamed by traditional research approaches which aim to collect information in a linear, systematic and controlled way. Such approaches, which are hierarchically created and defended by scientists, aim to collapse patients' complex psychological worlds into a range of predictable indicators. However, none of these measures appear to be capable of conveying the total 'reality' of living with diabetes. As a result, the management of patients' worries remains messy – a paradox that results from the uncertainty and concomitant anxiety that diabetes appears to bring. Strangely, no one has actually looked at how patients marry all of these 'bits and pieces' together in a common-sense way so that they can survive the ordeal of diabetes.

Let us now look at the issue from a complexity perspective and see if this changes anything.

Complexity dynamics in the diabetes psychological world

Complexity essentially represents a more inclusive theory of how life 'is', encompassing the orderly and rational along with the unpredictable and disorderly. From this perspective, patients' stories provide novel and important insights into the 'mind games' that the diagnosis of a chronic disease can induce. Zoe Mendelson, an artist and writer diagnosed with type 1 diabetes in early adulthood, published a diary reflecting upon her personal journey. In her final discourse she wrote about her personal acceptance of the disease:

> For four years I have hoped each morning to wake up and be freed from the mundane pursuit of pursuing perfect blood glucose levels and the threat of slipping up with my health; to be rid of the hypos and hypers; to be unchained from my over-sized handbag full of NHS-draining equipment. Instead, at nearly 30, I find a new liberation: I am freed now from the wishfulness. Ordinary life is diabetes.[16]

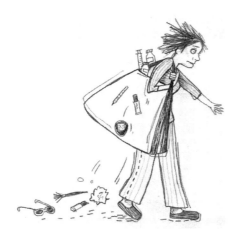

Throughout her diary she depicts a journey that was rich in learning, often in an unintended manner. The journey required continual self-organisation, new skills to deal with the paradoxes associated with living with a disease, continual learning from experience, and finally the emergence of a whole new mental approach to living with diabetes whereby she no longer questioned its boundaries. All of these are features of complex systems, and from this perspective, using our complexity mapping from the previous chapter, we can create a general picture of the psychological effects that diabetes can have on the individual – effects which can also be felt by those who live with and care for them.

Again, as we have seen in previous chapters, all of this makes reasonable sense. You would struggle to find a psychologist who wouldn't agree with the complex nature of the psychology of diabetes. However, because of the dominant orderly framework, most academic studies concentrate on just two aspects of diabetes – blood glucose control and quality of life – the bits it can accurately study. Alongside this,

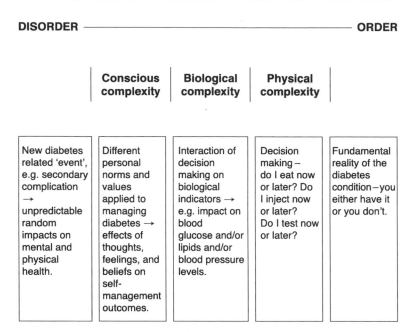

Figure 4.1: A complexity view of the psychology of diabetes.

government/health systems only put in minimal resources because the complex nature of diabetes psychology makes it extremely difficult to demonstrate the impact of those resources and therefore to justify their allocation against other resource demands. This inability to prove the impact of psychological interventions, yet common-sense recognition of their importance, lies at the heart of diabetes policy/practice paradoxes.

Another way of understanding the paradox: X–Y graphs vs. fitness landscapes

A classic mental model from an orderly perspective is the standard X–Y graph. The history of the graph goes back several centuries and passes through several cultures. In our case, it becomes firmly established through the work of Newton and Descartes. Descartes was so important in its development that points on the X–Y graph are still referred to as Cartesian coordinates. With an X–Y graph, any point on a two-dimensional surface can be plotted and connected. For orderly-based thinkers, the person with diabetes and the process of diabetes could be represented by the following graph.

From an orderly mechanistic perspective, the approach to the person with diabetes is to get them to move from point A to point B as quickly as possible, and then to keep them moving along from point B to point C for the foreseeable future. From this perspective, the goal is to get to point B as fast as possible and to remain stable at that level for as long as possible. This type of perspective is exactly what many policy actors want to see, because it is easy to follow the progress of any given patient (from their position on the graph), easy to calculate where the average patient is on the graph, and

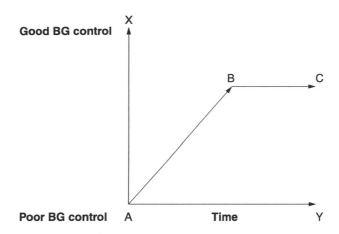

Figure 4.2: The orderly X–Y graph.

easy to judge how efficient any given hospital or treatment centre is (by simply comparing where all of their patients are in relation to the average patient position or in relation to set targets). All of this should sound horribly familiar, since it is being done throughout the health and education sectors. However, this perspective has several disturbing implications.

- There is an end point B. The goal is to get there fast and stay there. Any strategy that gets the patient to B faster must be better. Any strategy that keeps them on the B to C line longer must be better.
- Experts know how to get patients from A to B. They have seen many others get there, so the key is to do what the expert says (what others have done) and get to B as fast as possible. Once the patient is there, they should be encouraged to do exactly as they have done before, as this is the most likely strategy for keeping them on the line from B to C.
- Patients, due to their lack of knowledge, must be fundamentally passive, rely on experts and do as they are told. Carers must help to enforce these tactics.
- For patients and experts, diabetes management is basically a matter of repetition. If something goes wrong, repeat previous successful strategies. Experimentation, exploration and learning are best avoided and used only as a last resort.
- In general, for patients, non-control (failing to move quickly from A to B or falling off the B to C line) equals a 'lack of control' or failure to follow the rules. It is intrinsically the patient's fault. Experts are not responsible in such cases. One patient summarised this as follows:

> They'd look at your face and it was just like a road map and they'd . . . pick up on all the things and say, 'I know what you've been doing.' I used to find it quite demoralising because you are sitting there thinking, 'I am doing all right but maybe I'm not doing as well as I might.' With all due respect to them, they are very busy people, they don't have the time to sit and give you an individual conference even though that's really what this check-up is about and they have to be precious with their time. What you're doing then is you are condensing a bit of information about you into five or six

minutes that you are in there, and I always used to feel that, like, you were getting caught out. That's the feeling, it's like, I know I've been naughty but don't make me feel bad about it because I feel bad enough as it is.[17]

The image that the X–Y graph conjures up in the mind is that diabetes is like walking up a steep mountain. The expert is there to guide you up the mountain of control as quickly and efficiently as possible. Once you reach the top, the peak of control, there is nowhere else to go except to hold still. Any movement off the peak implies failure, mistakes and/or lack of control. The anxiety that is created by this desperate struggle to stay still through the normal bumpy ride of life is obviously enormous.

A different point of view: the fitness landscape

For simple orderly phenomena and systems, the X–Y graph is an excellent tool. To calculate the movements of balls on a table, the trajectory of missiles, etc. the X–Y graph is all you need. However, for complex systems you need a way of modelling and imagining a system that can move in varying and unpredictable ways over time. You need a way to show the probability of a system moving in a multitude of directions, a way to show how the system 'fits' with varying situations and circumstances. You need a fitness landscape.

Fitness landscapes were originally designed to model chemical and species interactions,[18] and are mathematically represented on a three-dimensional graph as follows.

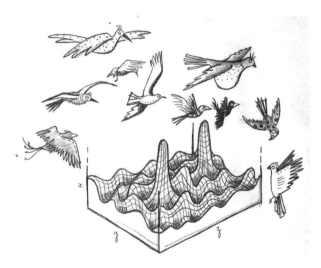

In these pictures, valleys represent areas of poor fitness, mountains represent areas of high fitness, and flatlands represent areas of neutral fitness. In other words, complex systems – such as schools of fish, herds of buffalo or entire species – are constantly moving through an evolving fitness landscape where new predators, food sources and numerous other factors combine to influence their chances of survival. Some of the basic rules of survival on a fitness landscape are adaptability, flexibility, learning and balance. So long as the 'system' survives, the fitness landscape continues to evolve through time like a never-ending conveyor belt.

Obviously, it doesn't take much of an imaginary leap to see how fitness landscapes would relate to diabetes. First, imagine a landscape that is full of flatlands, valleys and mountains and that stretches endlessly into the future. Now imagine that the valleys represent zones of poor control, the mountains represent zones of good control and the flatlands represent areas of uneven control. The important thing to note is that this does not produce a single mountain or a continuous mountain range surrounded by valleys. This is just another version of our orderly world view.

Instead, imagine a landscape where a number of mountains, flatlands and occasional valleys are clustered straight ahead of you. On either side, the mountains begin to shrink and become less frequent, the flatlands are fewer, and the valleys are more numerous and deeper.

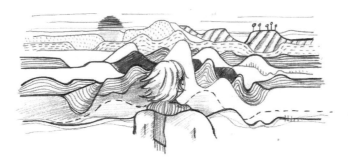

This is a good image of the fitness landscape for the average person with diabetes. Straight ahead is the path of reasonable strategies – good diet, regular exercise, balanced insulin usage, etc. This zone has many mountains of good fitness, but these don't stay the same all of the time. They are clustered in the reasonable strategies zone because these strategies are the most likely to produce good balance, but hidden valleys abound. A stressful period, hormonal changes, pregnancy and other significant life events all mask hidden valleys that a strict adherence to previous strategies cannot solve. On either side of the zone of reasonable strategies lie increasingly uncertain areas of deep and frequent valleys of poor balance, and only occasional mountains. As this image implies, life is tougher in these areas. For most people with diabetes, good balance is more difficult to maintain in these zones, but mountains of good balance do exist. Alcoholics or smokers may choose to live out in these more difficult zones. And people with unstable diabetes are often forced to travel through them.

Just as with species evolving through time, the primary tactics of people with diabetes travelling through their fitness landscape are adaptability, flexibility, learning and balance. In contrast to our orderly vision of a walk to the mountain top of control, a trek through the fitness landscape of diabetes reveals a number of remarkable 'common-sense' implications.

- There is no end point to a fitness landscape, nor is there any final resting point. The primary goal and tactic is adaptation and balance to changing circumstances.
- The main actor on treks across the fitness landscape is *you*. You are actively moving through the landscape. You make essential choices. Your opinions, experiences and learning matter.

- Learning is essential and it never stops. Being aware, making choices, experimenting and exploring is how you learn about your landscape and evolve personal tactics for dealing with the inevitable unknown.
- Experts are helpers on your journey. Their advice is important, but ultimately you decide.
- Change is not bad. You are not desperately struggling to cling to a mountain top hoping that the next wind won't blow you off. You are learning a new way of living that offers a whole range of problems and challenges. Change is part of that world. Exploring and accepting that change is what makes it all worthwhile.
- As you explore, mistakes, misdirections and occasional stumbles into valleys are *normal* and are not a mark of weakness or failure. The only mistake is refusing to see them as normal and not learning from them.

Fundamentally, a trek through the fitness landscape is very similar to the concept of 'transformative learning.' This is defined as learning that involves:

> experiencing a deep, structural shift in basic premises of thought, feelings and actions. It is a shift of consciousness that dramatically and permanently alters our way of being in the world.[19]

This was translated unintentionally by Zoe Mendelson when she wrote:

> Could my life actually be fuller and richer than it would have been without diabetes? . . . There is, of course, the possibility that I have done more than I would have done had I not felt that an obstacle to my potential had been lodged in my path.

However, the question remains, how does one reach this point?

Learning about yourself: losing the anxiety

From the traditional perspective, there is growing evidence that psychological counselling can contribute to 'improved adherence and psychological outcomes in people with diabetes.'[20] It is interesting to note the continuation of the relationship between psychological outcomes and blood glucose control, now addressed in the medical literature as 'adherence.' We know, however, that there is a lack of psychological help available in the health service, and that diabetes-related anxieties are common among patients. The implication is that too many people trap themselves on a mountain top, desperately afraid of change, adaptation and learning, resulting in unnecessary anxiety, stress and depression.

Can patient education make a difference?

Recent international initiatives are aiming to change these patterns through the process of patient education. There are a wide variety of diabetes education initiatives throughout the world. Unfortunately, but not surprisingly, most of these have taken a top-down approach with professionals dominating the learning process (thereby downplaying patient expertise), a focus on 'control' with scant attention to what may really matter to patients, and separation of the learning process into discrete bits and pieces, thereby losing the multifaceted nature of learning how to live with diabetes in the real world. Not surprisingly, given these limitations, a recent systematic review of existing diabetes patient educational interventions found insufficient evidence available to recommend a specific type of education or provide guidance on the setting or frequency of sessions. However, there are some exceptions to this. For example, research conducted in the UK summarised what patients valued most about education[21] (*see* Box 4.1). To be successful, it highlighted the need to integrate personal experiences into the educational process. This method acknowledges the expertise that patients develop from living with their diabetes. It affirms the belief that besides formal learning there is an even greater amount of learning that can result from everyday experiences. Learning is therefore achieved by making new information meaningful to patients by relating it to *their* life experiences, *their* emotional feelings and *their* feelings about what will happen if they do or do not follow the 'rules.' This is what adult education is all about, because it has personal meaning and as such can contribute toward the journey of transformative learning. The emphasis here is on the word 'journey', but perhaps 'expedition' would be a more appropriate term for some!

Box 4.1: Summary of what patients value about education

- Protected time for learning and for reflection on learning: time for reappraisal to clarify and interpret the complexities of diabetes self-management.
- Augmentation of prior knowledge: new information and experiences integrated with existing knowledge and experiences.
- Collaborative approach to learning between patient and 'teacher', with personal experiences valued and likened to expertise.
- Learner-centred approach using principles of adult education.
- Supportive environment created by peer learning, allowing shared empathy for difficulties encountered in the 'real world', and increased motivation.

An old approach from a different perspective

Given this educational perspective, the traditional research approach of reducing the 'mind games' associated with learning how to live with diabetes into separate psychological categories appears restrictive and illogical. History tells us that it has served only to fragment what is a way of life for many people, and reflects a growing trend in our society towards reducing problems that are essentially non-reducible. This implies that complexity is more aligned to 'real life' with diabetes. It draws together all of the different factors, creating a common-sense patchwork, and highlights the simple fact that change is a normal part of our lives. Just knowing this may help in responding to uncertainty, because with change comes the need for continual adaptation and exploration and hence necessary mistakes. Thus there may be partial order and partial disorder, predictability and probability but also uncertainty. Essentially the processes are about emergence, innovation, learning and adaptation.[20] As Geyer[22] has indicated, complexity is a framework of thinking that gives a larger scientific foundation to daily common-sense strategies, rather than a magic wand for perfectly solving them. From this perspective there are therefore no quick fixes. Just as with any changes in life, adjustment will take a variable length of time. It is essentially a journey and, like any journey where we are not too sure where we are going, we need a personal map. Some will require assistance to navigate this map, while others may get there on their own. Either way, the destination is a place where the mind games become a normal part of the person living with diabetes, so that the disease and all that it brings become an ordinary way of life, not just for the patient but for those around him or her.

An old Chinese proverb perhaps neatly summarises these thoughts. See what you think:

> A reed cannot change its place in the field, but can only learn to move and bend with the changing elements.

Another silly exercise

Take a piece of A4 paper and crumple it into a ball. Then unwrap it and flatten it out on a table in front of you. Don't flatten it completely – allow it to remain crumpled. At the bottom of the paper write 'Now' and at the top write 'The Future.' On the left-hand side write 'Diabetes.' Circle some of the mountains and valleys on the paper and ask yourself what circumstances might lead you to a new mountain peak of high 'fitness' or into a new valley of low 'fitness.' In many cases, these may be the same events for people with diabetes. A new job or relationship might give you the confidence to reach a new peak or add a new type of stress that pushes you into a valley. On the other hand, a new setback, job loss or crisis at work may shove you into a valley, but may also be the path to a new mountain. Such events may also impact upon carers and health professionals and their relationships with the person who has diabetes. As with our last exercise, there is no right or wrong answer. It is just a way of showing that we are all, whether we have diabetes or not, on our own trek on the fitness landscape. Learning, exploring, adapting and accepting are what it is all about. Read Kathleen's story as she 'looks back', and see if you can relate to what she has discovered.

Looking back . . . Kathleen's story

> I have lived with diabetes for a long time. As I look back I can think of a number of incidents which propelled me toward acceptance of my disease so that it became a part of me. Some are normal life things that many people experience – leaving home, going to university, getting married, having children, starting a new job. But there are others which are quite unique to having a disease, many of which were small in their own way but had huge effects – experiencing a severe hypo, a doctor asking the right question at the right time, meeting others with diabetes, realising that diabetes can actually lead to loss of vision, kidney failure and other 'nasties.' I could go on, but what I know is that whilst a 'grief reaction' happened, it was overlaid by an ordinary life in which these events occurred, which is why I can talk about normal life-changing events such as getting married and having children.

> What was my 'grief reaction' then? Did it follow the pattern so well documented as a process of feeling hopeless and helpless, of questioning

'Why me?', of anger and denial? As I look back the answer has to be yes, but it was also much more than this. It didn't just 'happen' as an event, but it was spread out over a long period of time. It was gradual and, as such, I did have feelings of sadness and helplessness, but these times were interwoven with long periods of satisfaction and happiness, or just feeling OK. What was important were the people who surrounded me who unconsciously treated me like everybody else, thus providing the setting for a relatively normal life. Just like everyone else, but with different life challenges. Perhaps the most important point came when I realised that I could not expect others to truly understand because they do not have the disease and, as such, it was mine to manage and mine to control. I had a responsibility not just to myself but to others around me. Diabetes therefore became a piece of me – a lifelong companion. It is no longer an alien, obtrusive part of my life. It just is. The mind games will never stop because diabetes will always be with me, but the games now end quickly and I always seem to win! The anxiety has gone, to be replaced by a kind of inner peace. The restrictions now seem perfectly normal. The beauty of all this is that the lessons I have learned from living with diabetes apply to so many other parts of my life.

References

1 Lennon J. *The John Lennon Collection*. London: EMI Records Ltd; 1982.
2 Kutchins H, Kirk SA. *Making us Crazy*. London: Constable; 1999. p. 22.
3 Anderson RJ, Freedland KE, Clouse RE *et al*. The prevalence of comorbid depression in adults with diabetes: a meta-analysis. *Diabetes Care*. 2001; **24**: 1069–78.
4 Grigsby AB, Anderson RJ, Freedland KE *et al*. Prevalence of anxiety in adults with diabetes: a systematic review. *J Psychosom Res*. 2002; **53**: 1053–60.
5 Lin EH, Katon W, Von Korff M *et al*. Relationship of depression and diabetes self-care, medication adherence, and preventive care. *Diabetes Care*. 2004; **27**: 2154–60.
6 De Groot M, Anderson R, Freedland KE *et al*. Association of depression and diabetes complications: a meta-analysis. *Psychosom Med*. 2001; **63**: 619–30.
7 Gede LE, Zheng P, Simpson K. Comorbid depression is associated with increased health care use and expenditures in individuals with diabetes. *Diabetes Care*. 2002; **25**: 464–70.
8 Department of Health and Diabetes UK. *Structured Patient Education in Diabetes: report from the Patient Education Working Group*. London: Department of Health Publications; 2005.
9 Dunn SM, Turtle J. The myth of the diabetic personality. *Diabetes Care*. 1981; **4**: 640–46.
10 Hayes M. A phenomenological study of chronic sorrow in people with type 1 diabetes. *Pract Diabetes Int*. 2001; **18**: 65–9.
11 Polly RK. Diabetes health beliefs, self-care behaviors, and glycaemic control among older adults with non-insulin-dependent diabetes mellitus. *Diabetes Educator*. 1992; **18**: 321–7.
12 Dunn SM. Reactions to educational techniques: coping strategies for diabetes and learning. *Diabet Med*. 1986; **3**: 419–29.
13 Hampson HE, Glasgow RE, Toobert DJ. Personal models of diabetes and their relations to self-care activities. *Health Psychol*. 1990; **9**: 632–46.
14 Bradley C, editor. *Handbook of Psychology and Diabetes*. Chur, Switzerland: Harwood Academic Publishers; 1994.
15 Peyrot M, Runib RR, Lauritzen FJ *et al*. Psychosocial problems and barriers to improved diabetes management: results of the cross-national diabetes attitudes. Diabetes Attitudes, Wishes and Needs (DAWN) Study. *Diabet Med*. 2005; **22**: 1379–85.
16 Mendleson Z. I'm faring well. *Balance*. 2005; **207**: 7.

17 Cooper H. *Capturing the impact of patient education on people with type 2 diabetes.* Unpublished PhD thesis. Liverpool: University of Liverpool; 2001.

18 Gell-Mann M. *The Quark and the Jaguar: adventures in the simple and complex.* New York: WH Freeman and Co.; 1994.

19 *Transformative Learning Centre;* www.oise.utoronto.ca/~tlcentre/index.htm (accessed January 2005).

20 International Diabetes Federation. *Global Guideline for Type 2 Diabetes: psychological care;* www.idf.org/webdata/docs/GGT2D%2004%20Psychological%20care.pdf (accessed January 2006).

21 Cooper H, Booth K, Gill G. Patients' perspectives on diabetes health care education. *Health Educ Res.* 2003; **18:** 191–206.

22 Geyer R. Beyond the Third Way: the science of complexity and the politics of choice. *Br J Politics Int Relations.* 2003; **5:** 237–57.

Chapter 5

Managing the complexities of diabetes

If things were that simple, word would have gotten round.

Jacques Derrida (famous French philosopher)

What would you do with a brain if you had one?

Dorothy speaking to the Scarecrow in *The Wizard of Oz*

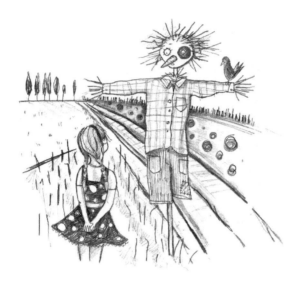

These two quotes neatly capture the two underlying lessons of this chapter. First, that despite the hopes and dreams of traditional mechanistic science, life – and diabetes – just aren't that simple. If they were, as Derrida tells us, 'word would have gotten round.' Not only are these dreams of order unrealistic, but if you think about it for a minute you will realise that life wouldn't be the same without its joyous complexity. Uncertainty, unpredictability, change and learning are built into our lives and help to make up the breadth of the human experience. The complexity of the diabetes experience mirrors life's reality.

Secondly, as most of us remember in *The Wizard of Oz*, Dorothy picks up three companions – the Scarecrow, the Tin Man and the Lion – on the way to the Emerald City. Each of them feels they are missing something. The Scarecrow, with his head of straw, feels that he is lacking a brain, and heads off with the others to see the Wizard of Oz to seek one. As the story continues, the Scarecrow makes a number of key decisions that save the day, and eventually devises a plan to save Dorothy from the Wicked Witch. In the end, after going through the adventure, the Scarecrow realises that he has a brain after all. Like the Scarecrow, diabetes raises the need for a 'brain' to deal with its unpredictable nature. In reality, however, we all have a range of complex experiences to draw upon to help us to do this so that, like the Scarecrow, we are already experts at dealing with 'complex situations', often without realising it. Dealing with diabetes therefore expands this expertise. After all, would the Scarecrow have been so smart if someone had solved his problems for him? In essence, this takes us back to Dorothy's question, 'What would you do with a brain if you had one?'

Why is management complex?

As we saw in the last chapter, experts may understand the general picture, but patients know about 'living' with the disease on a day-to-day basis. People with diabetes inevitably acquire knowledge and experience of their condition and its management, and therefore become experts in living with their disease. In the same way, health professionals and those who live with patients develop knowledge and experience relative to the roles they play in the lives of patients. Marrying all of these individual views together to find acceptable strategies for management can be a tricky business. In some situations, simple mechanistic rules may apply. For example, where diabetes control is adequate, exercise will reduce blood glucose levels and therefore more carbohydrate intake and/or less insulin is required. Or, in an emergency situation such as diabetic ketoacidosis or severe hypoglycaemia, an immediate expert response may make the difference between life and death. However, there are many situations where the answers are far from certain and there is little agreement about how the patient should be managed. For example, managing the vagaries of so-called 'brittle' or unstable diabetes requires much more than just 'standard responses.' It demands creativity, intuition and experimentation in an attempt to find things that work for the individual patient. More commonly, even simple decisions about the best strategies for encouraging weight loss may be fraught with hidden complexities.

The art of management: from hierarchical to interactive management

Most of us, when we think of management, think of the traditional top-down, 'command-and-control', hierarchical type of management typified by large corporations, government bureaucracies and the military. In these cases, knowledge, control and decision making rest with elites at the top of a hierarchy. It is the job of those lower in the hierarchy to do as they are told as thoroughly and completely as possible, and to relay information up the chain of command to enable those at the top to make appropriate decisions.

The foundation of this style of management is the orderly mechanistic framework of Newton and Descartes. This type of so-called 'scientific management' assumes that there is clear cause and effect, predictability and determinism. It presupposes that those at the top know all of the relevant information and what is best for the company, bureaucracy or army as a whole. Elites in this type of system are almost demi-gods, and are often given the lofty title, salary and prestige that reflect such exalted positions, and they have an obvious interest in maintaining the system. Many non-elites are very supportive of this system as well. They can ignore problems and complications because they are 'doing as they are told', and all the while they are free from the burden of responsibility. For much of the twentieth century, this was the dominant form of managerial thinking.

However, from the mid-twentieth century onward more and more people began to question the dominance of this type of management thinking. Some noted that elites never had all the information and weren't always acting in the best interest of the company, department, etc. Others saw that this radically stifled the potential of non-elites to solve local problems and issues. As we have seen earlier, this type of management works for simple problems and issues, but comes unstuck in the face of the complexity of daily life. Unsurprisingly, in the last 10 to 20 years complexity has been acting as a foundation for a whole new way of looking at management.

The leader in this field is Professor Ralph Stacey from the University of Hertford-shire, who has written a huge range of books and articles. One of the most useful concepts that he developed was what we will call the *Stacey diagram*. In this remarkably simple yet powerful diagram, Stacey combined two different aspects – the *degree of certainty* and the *level of agreement* – to demonstrate a whole range of complex everyday decision making.

The Stacey diagram: what does it look like?

To build a Stacey diagram you start with a typical two dimensional X–Y diagram. Each axis is given one aspect. The degree of certainty is put on the horizontal axis, and the level of agreement on the vertical axis, as shown below.

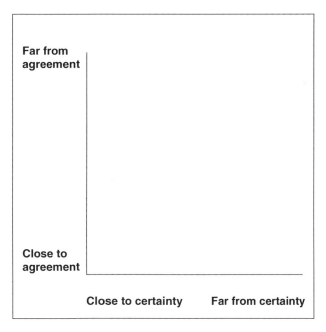

Figure 5.1: Stacey diagram 1.

Now what did Stacey mean by each of these dimensions?

The 'certainty dimension'

Close to certainty

Issues or decisions are close to certainty when cause and effect are known. This is usually the case when we are faced with a familiar situation, and it is the essence of experiential learning. We tend to use the same actions as before, with the knowledge that they will work. For example, to rectify hypoglycaemia, the administration of quick-acting sugar in the form of glucose is advised.

Far from certainty

At the other end are decisions that are far from certainty. These situations are often unique or at least new to us, so that we have no prior experiences that we can use to predict outcomes. The cause and effect linkages are therefore not clear. For example, for a teenager with diabetes who is self-harming himself, the exact role that diabetes is playing in this behaviour is very far from certain.

The 'agreement dimension'

Close to agreement

These are decisions where all of the actors involved agree on the nature and type of decision. For example, there is generally little debate between patients with type 1 diabetes and health professionals that they need insulin on a regular basis, or for that matter that they need to eat a balanced diet.

Far from agreement

In this area, there is little agreement between the actors on the nature and type of decision. This can take a variety of forms. It may be a disagreement between experts over the effectiveness of certain treatments, between the patient and the doctor about acceptable eating behaviour, or between the patient and the carer about the need to adhere to the 'rules.'

By bringing these dimensions together, Stacey highlighted five different zones which he illustrated graphically:

- *zone 1* – close to agreement, close to certainty
- *zone 2* – far from agreement, close to certainty
- *zone 3* – close to agreement, far from certainty
- *zone 4* – far from agreement, far from certainty
- *zone 5* – mixed agreement and certainty.

These zones are not dissimilar to the five boxes discussed in Chapter 3. In many ways they represent a similar range of processes applied to decision making. But what are these zones and how do they relate to diabetes management?

Zone 1 – close to agreement, close to certainty: the zone of the technical expert

This region, where the problem and the response are clear and actors agree on how the problem should be solved, is the zone of the technical expert. If you fall and have a

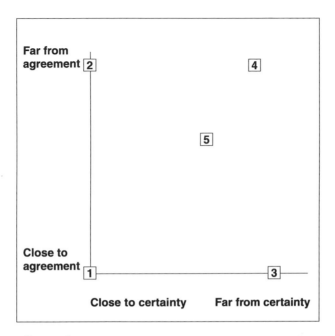

Figure 5.2: Stacey diagram 2.

simple leg fracture, all experts agree that the leg should be reset in a plaster cast, and you are very unlikely to disagree with them. In general, this zone tends to be where actions and decisions are based on past experiences. In other words, we gather data

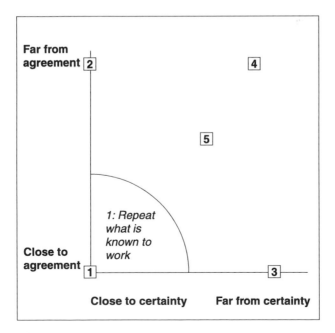

Figure 5.3: Stacey diagram 3.

from the past and use this to predict the future. Evidence-based medicine falls neatly into this zone. An example is the treatment of mild hypoglycaemia. Taking three glucose sweets usually returns blood glucose levels to normal pretty quickly. Following this with some complex carbohydrate such as a banana or an oat biscuit will usually prevent hypoglycaemia occurring again before the next meal or snack. All experts agree on this response, and most patients would not find this a difficult procedure to follow.

Zone 2 – far from agreement, close to certainty: the zone of 'political' decisions

Some issues have a great deal of certainty about how outcomes are created, but high levels of disagreement about which outcomes are desirable. These issues are more complicated and are very similar to the 'political' issues that are continually debated in society and within families. In this context, individual views are important. In the medical consultation, such situations require negotiation and compromise. For example, when blood glucose levels are inadequately controlled, the doctor or nurse may suggest changes in lifestyle to tackle not only blood glucose levels but also excess weight. Patients may not dispute the outcomes of poor control, but they may disagree with the expert over strategies. Both parties have their own agendas (which are far from agreement) – for the patient it is about maintaining the status quo of their

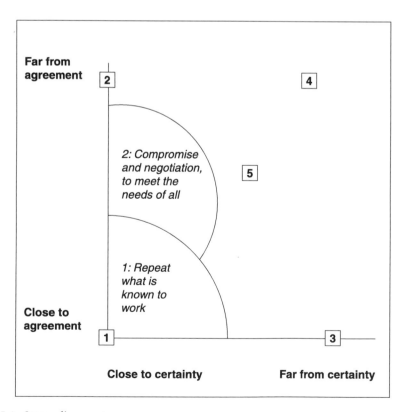

Figure 5.4: Stacey diagram 4.

lifestyle, whereas for the doctor or nurse it is about reaching targets that are known to prevent complications. Both relate to quality of life (close to certainty). Negotiation is therefore required to reach some sort of agreement about how blood glucose levels can be balanced.

Zone 3 – close to agreement, far from certainty: the zone of judgemental decisions

Some issues have a high level of agreement but not much certainty as to how to make them happen – that is, the outcomes are clear but the means of getting there are not. The cause and effect linkages are therefore unknown. In this second complicated zone, the goal is to move towards an agreed upon future state using judgement, even though the specific paths for getting there are not yet clear. Both experts and patients have an important role to play in this zone. For example, everybody agrees that the responsibility for diabetes management ultimately resides with the patient, but the means of getting the majority of patients to do this successfully are not clearly understood. For instance, a patient and carer may agree that it is in the best interests of the patient to lose weight, but the way to achieve this weight loss is often far from certain. Judgemental decisions based on an ongoing patient–carer dialogue are the best way forward.

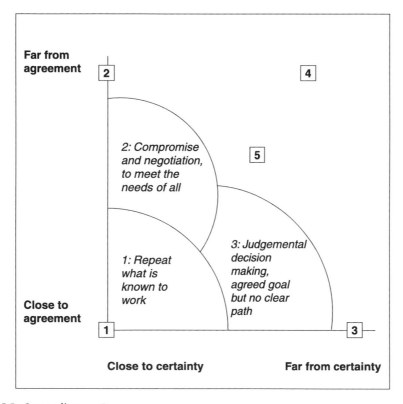

Figure 5.5: Stacey diagram 5.

Health professionals and patients spend much of their time in zones 1, 2 and 3, and evidence-based medicine sits neatly in these three areas. In many ways, these three zones are understandable from a traditional mechanical perspective – medical research is all about pushing more aspects of diabetes management into zone 1 and out of zones 2 and 3. However, as we have seen all along, health is much more than a mechanical process.

Zone 4 – far from agreement, far from certainty: the zone of disorder

Looking at the opposite end of the spectrum, some issues have very high levels of uncertainty and disagreement. These situations are the most unpredictable and can be the most difficult to deal with. The traditional methods of planning and negotiation are inadequate, and people often deal with such situations by 'muddling through' or avoidance. Both of these approaches are probably protective strategies in the short term, but they can be disastrous in the long term. For example, a newly diagnosed adolescent patient who denies his diabetes and ignores the 'rules' is far from agreement about his new-found condition and far from certain about what he should do about things. Denial is a common route. He goes out late and drinks alcohol to excess, which results in severe hypoglycaemia and hospital admission. Another example would be the patient with so-called unstable or 'brittle' diabetes.

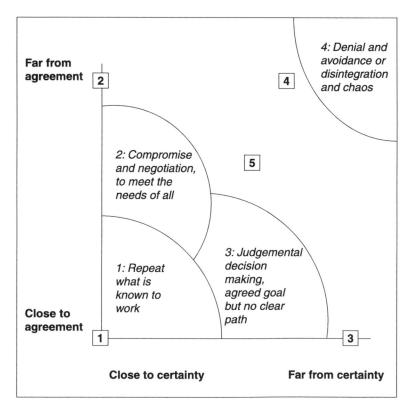

Figure 5.6: Stacey diagram 6.

Obviously this can be a very dangerous zone of uncertainty. But is this zone so uncommon in our daily lives? For example, choosing a life partner is one of the most uncertain and 'far from agreement' long-term decisions that can be made. An 'expert' opinion would only be of marginal use. Yet we do it all the time, and mostly reasonable outcomes occur, although about half of all life partnerships now fail. In this zone, muddling through is about the best we can do. Ignoring and denying the reality of this zone do not make it go away!

Zone 5 – mixed certainty/agreement: the zone of complexity and learning

This zone lies between the regions of chaos and traditional management approaches. In previous chapters, we have called this region the zone of complexity and used the middle three boxes as an illustration. In this region, traditional management approaches are not very effective, so it is the zone where people need to learn new approaches and new techniques, and maybe even unlearn tried and tested methods. This zone requires a range of approaches to deal with complex situations. Some of these approaches will have no evidence base but will be based on expert opinion or on intuition. For example, this is the researcher's world, where they test out new ideas, many of which are based on observation. It is the area where new treatments are

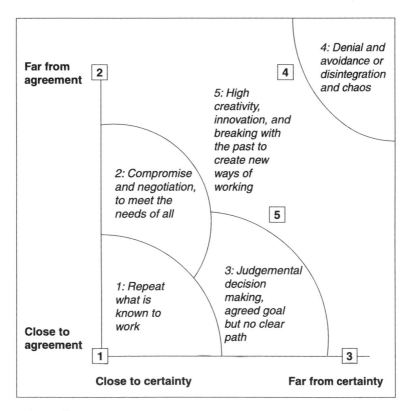

Figure 5.7: Stacey diagram 7.

discovered, such as inhaled insulin, where DAFNE and DESMOND education programmes were devised, and where insulin was first discovered. It is also the region where patients experiment – learning how to adjust insulin dosages to meet the demands of a changing lifestyle, testing out the effects of different foods on blood glucose levels, and finding out what can happen if the rules are 'broken.' For the adolescent newly diagnosed with diabetes, it is the time when he has to face up to being 'different' to his peers and find new ways of coping. It can be a difficult time, a time when 'mind games' predominate, but as was discussed in the last chapter, it is also a time for new and transformative learning.

Have a go

Now that Stacey's five zones have been described, try having a go yourself. Take a piece of paper and a pen. Write down any issues/questions that come to mind about diabetes – you can write anything. Now, using a simplified version of the Stacey diagram as shown below, see whether you can decide which of the five zones your issues/questions fit into. Some may fit into more than one zone. As in earlier chapters, this is not just an exercise for patients. Experts in diabetes and carers should try to play this game as well. Ideally, patients, experts and carers should play this game together and use the diagram as a way of understanding and coming to terms with a particular

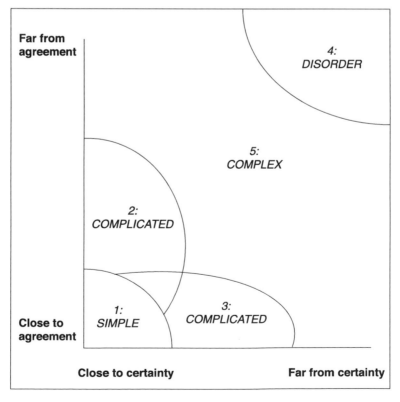

Figure 5.8: Stacey diagram 8.

treatment or aspect of diabetes. The diagram will not solve problems, but it may help you to understand the nature of those problems and the kind of response necessary, and it may help you to communicate your understanding to the other players (carers, experts, family, etc.).

You will probably find that some of your issues/questions have fallen into zone 5, the complexity/learning zone. These types of issues/questions are what you might call 'tricky' (others call them 'wicked') because they are complex and, from your perspective, they appear to have no clear answers. For example, 'Will diabetes ever be cured?' The answer is obviously impossible to predict – we have to wait for it to emerge through the development of new ideas. A similar question is 'How long will I live with diabetes?' Other things that you have written may have fallen into zones 2 and/or 3, complicated questions for which there are no simple answers. For example, the constant pull between wants and desires, and the nagging question of whether or not you should give in are a daily challenge. The answer probably depends upon compromise and negotiation with yourself, whether you have diabetes or not! Other questions may fall into zone 1 because the answers are more clear-cut – for example, 'What cholesterol levels should I aim for?', 'How much alcohol can I safely drink?', 'Do I take my insulin when I am unwell and not eating much?' The answers to these questions are relatively simple because the cause and effect linkages are known – they have a strong evidence base as a result of rigorous research (see www.diabetes.org.uk for answers).

You may now feel that this exercise has provided a framework to help you rationalise some of your feelings and actions. Just like complexity mapping, the fitness landscape, the Stacey diagram and the complexity cascade (which we shall explore in the next chapter) all serve to reinforce the fact that learning how to manage different situations or issues requires you to get a feel for what type of problem/question you are trying to address and then respond to it in a reasonably appropriate fashion. Please note that there are no clear boundaries between zones, and one person's 'political' decision may be another's technical one. Continual learning, exploring, adapting and accepting of what comes your way are the only long-term certainties that you have. As you learn more, through experience, reading or talking to others, some of your issues/questions will move from one zone to another. The next section of this chapter illustrates just this. It provides an example of a question that fell into zone 5, and it shows how creativity was used to provide an answer.

The diabetes boxes: going three-dimensional

A question that fell into zone 5 for one of the authors of this book (Helen Cooper) was how to help people of all ages who have diabetes to understand and communicate what is happening to them. Locked into a strange new world, beset by often overwhelming complexities, and sometimes even lacking a language in which to articulate what they are feeling, a diabetes diagnosis can lead to all sorts of problems, particularly emotional ones. Promoting understanding and communication is therefore extremely important for all involved – patients, carers and professionals. Unfortunately, much of what we know about diabetes relates to theories and biological concepts that can be difficult for people to grasp. Creativity and complexity thinking provided a way forward. The need to explore new ways to help people learn led to the design of interactive consulting and learning aids, designed with an artist (Alison Jones from Pioneer Projects) in the form of three 'Diabetes Boxes' (*see* Figure 5.9). Each box – a three-dimensional hand-made cube – is used to stimulate discussion, to help people to develop knowledge and understanding of the biological and psychological concepts relating to diabetes, and to help them to understand and express their feelings about having the disease.[1]

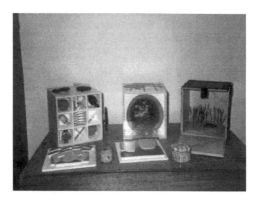

Figure 5.9: The diabetes boxes.

Each box relates to a specific theme.

Box 1: Why am I asked to make changes to my lifestyle? What am I trying to prevent?

This box depicts the difference between a healthy and an unhealthy (atherosclerotic) blood vessel. On one side of the box is a healthy artery, represented by a waterfall flowing through a round and clear 'vessel.' On the other side of the box is the unhealthy artery, represented by a stagnant stream running thorough a marsh, which ends up as a trickle of water coming out of a thickened 'vessel.' On all four sides of the box are images representing components of a healthy lifestyle that can minimise development of the unhealthy artery (i.e. exercise, diet, drug treatments and maintaining a balance). This box aims to help people to understand the reasoning behind treatment recommendations. To support this, two pots – one containing lard (slimy) and the other containing treacle (sticky) – are used alongside the box. Each person is asked to feel and describe the contents of the pots and then to relate this exercise to the box and its contents – in other words, to answer the question for themselves.

Box 2: What do I want to know about diabetes? What is important to me?

This box is used to generate discussion about a particular topic of interest or concern to the patient. One side of the box is divided into nine small compartments. Each compartment contains things that a person with diabetes has to remember to do, such as checking blood/urine glucose levels, taking medication and eating healthy foods. Centrally placed in the box is a coiled spring which represents different things to different people – for example, the tension created by living with diabetes until such practices become an accepted part of their life. The reverse side of this box has doors which open on to a three-dimensional image of a beach with waves, sand and shells. It is used to generate discussion on such issues as stress and its effects on blood glucose levels, the psychological processes associated with accepting diabetes, and the process of changing lifestyle behaviours. It aims to help people to talk about their personal concerns and their personal feelings.

Box 3: What can happen to me if I don't follow the 'rules'? What are my responsibilities?

This box relates to the long-term complications of diabetes and their relationship to screening, treatment and lifestyle. On the outside of the box are images representing the organs which can be potentially affected by the disease process – eyes, kidneys, heart, nerve fibres and feet. These can be used to generate discussion on screening procedures, patients' uncertainties and their personal responsibilities. The box collapses to reveal an image of a bed of reeds around a pool. This relates to the proverb previously quoted in Chapter 4:

> A reed cannot change its place in the field, but can only learn to move and bend with the changing elements.

This proverb links into the permanence of diabetes (the reed cannot change its place in the field) and the need to make changes (learn to bend with the changing elements) in order to minimise the consequences of the disease. Patients are asked to consider the link between the proverb and diabetes for themselves.

Outcomes

The boxes have proved to be very successful, generating a great deal of interest among both patients and professionals. Since they were originally produced, they have been replicated for others to use, they have been utilised to teach health professionals from a variety of disciplines, and they have also been reproduced for use with four different ethnic communities, each box being adapted to take into account cultural diversity (*see* Figures 5.10 and 5.11).[2]

Their success raises the question of how something so simple proved effective in addressing something so complex. The answer relates to complexity thinking. Although there was no clear evidence base for the boxes, the idea was based on expert intuition. Such intuition stemmed from the simple fact that living successfully with diabetes requires a great deal of learning – not just about its individual components but, more importantly, about how these components interact with and affect each other. The boxes empowered people to do this for themselves – to put it all together from their own personal perspective – and in so doing filled a gap that traditional practices had failed to fill in the past. As Einstein once said:

> To raise new questions, new possibilities, to regard old problems from a new angle requires creative imagination and marks real advances in science.

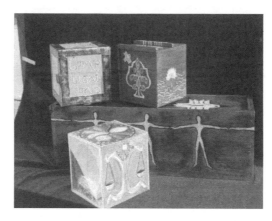

Figure 5.10: South Asian diabetes boxes.

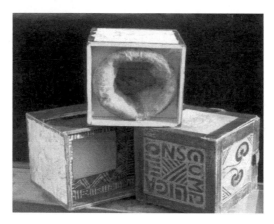

Figure 5.11: Afro-Caribbean diabetes boxes.

And the moral of this tale?

Art, it seems, has a place in the traditionally scientific, evidence-based world of medicine, particularly when the success of treatment depends upon patients' self-management practices and not just expert advice. In many ways, the boxes merely lift the process of complexity mapping off the written page and put them into patients' hands. As we have argued throughout this book, this provides a place where one can 'see' how all the bits and their interconnections fit together. In so doing, complexity makes sense of diabetes and its management and the need for a wide range of approaches, not all of which fit into the traditional medical evidence-based 'box.' In so doing, it recognises that going beyond traditional practices is not only acceptable but also essential.

One more thing

If you like the idea of the three-dimensional diabetes boxes, we encourage you to make your own, modelled on your particular needs or situation, or you can purchase copies of the ones shown here. The boxes can be made to fit your specific requirements by contacting Alison Jones at Pioneer Projects (www.pioneerprojects.org.uk).

References

1 Cooper H. LAY Foundations of diabetes care. *Pract Nurse J.* 1994; **7**: 78–82.
2 Cooper H, Jones A. Connecting art to health care education: evaluation of a project with ethnic minority groups in Liverpool. *Diab Med.* 2002; **19(suppl 2)**: A90: 23.

Further reading on the work of Ralph Stacey

Stacey R. *Managing the Unknowable: strategic boundaries between order and chaos in organizations.* San Francisco, CA: Jossey-Bass Publishers; 1992.

Stacey R. Emerging strategies for a chaotic environment. *Long-Range Planning.* 1996; **16**: 182–9.

Stacey R. *Strategic Management and Organisational Dynamics: the challenge of complexity.* 3rd ed. New York: Prentice Hall; 1999.

Stacey R, Griffin D, editors. *Complexity and the Experience of Managing in Public Sector Organisations.* London: Routledge; 2005.

Stacey R, Griffin D, Shaw P, editors. *Complexity and Management: fad or radical challenge to systems thinking?* London: Routledge; 2000.

Chapter 6

Diabetes and the 'cascade of complexity'

Studying complex systems 'is like walking through a maze whose walls rearrange themselves with each step you take.'

(James Gleick, *Chaos*)

Alice is asking directions from the Cheshire Cat in Lewis Carol's *Alice in Wonderland*.

'Would you tell me, please, which way I ought to go from here?'
'That depends a good deal on where you want to get to,' said the Cat.
'I don't much care where–' said Alice.
'Then it doesn't matter which way you go,' said the Cat.
'– so long as I get SOMEWHERE,' Alice added as an explanation.
'Oh, you're sure to do that,' said the Cat, 'if you only walk long enough.'

Despite being written in very different times and for very different audiences, these quotes nicely express the emergent, evolving and unpredictable nature of complexity and how the mind has to deal with it. And yet, signposts and practice can help us negotiate this ever-changing complexity maze and eventually get us SOMEWHERE.

In this chapter we want to introduce you to four more concepts from complexity and explore how they can help you to understand the nature of diabetes. These are:

- punctuated equilibrium
- frozen accidents
- regularities
- gateway events.

With these concepts we shall introduce and explore how they, you, life and diabetes fit into the *cascade of complexity*.

Punctuated equilibrium, frozen accidents, regularities and gateway events

To understand these concepts we must first return to our traditional orderly mechanistic framework and ask how change is supposed to occur in our traditional 'mechanical' world. Fundamentally, it is based on the concept of smooth transitions from one state to another, and the movement towards a final resting or 'equilibrium' state. The simplest and most classic example is the movement of a ball on the end of a string – a simple pendulum. Add energy by pushing it, and it will start to move at a steady pace, back and forth. As friction takes effect it will slow down and eventually stop, reaching its final resting place or point of equilibrium. This is the same as our X–Y graph in Chapter 4. The ideal patient moves smoothly from poor control to good control and stays there in the 'final resting place' (yes, a pun is intended) or point of equilibrium.

This concept of smooth movement towards equilibrium runs throughout the natural, health and social sciences. In biology, mechanistic interpretations of Darwinian theory saw the evolution of life on earth as a calm and stately development from 'lower' life forms to the highest life form, human beings. From this perspective it didn't take much of an intellectual leap to view humans racially along the same lines. This became the widespread science of eugenics that was popular in the late nineteenth and early twentieth centuries. If animals evolve smoothly from lowest to highest, then humans must do the same (evolving from 'backwards' non-white tribal peoples to 'advanced' white Anglo-Europeans). The parallel is obvious. From the mechanical perspective, with the evolution of 'advanced' human beings, evolution reached its point of final equilibrium of human superiority.[1]

Punctuated equilibrium

The problem with this is that evolution doesn't work that way. In general, biological systems remain relatively stable for long periods of time and then tend to undergo fast radical change. In other words, evolution wasn't a leisurely stroll to the present day, but a jerky pattern of stability and change. This interrupted pattern is referred to as *punctuated equilibrium*.[2] What this implies is that in the complex everyday world that we inhabit, smooth changes towards stable end states only happen in the most simple and orderly aspects of our lives. Moreover, as we have seen before, there is no final, stable equilibrium. Returning to the example of our X–Y graph, a more realistic, 'complex' interpretation of diabetes would look like the following.

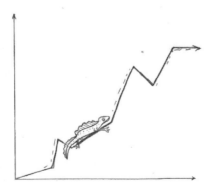

Frozen accidents

Building on the idea of punctuated equilibrium are the concepts of frozen accidents and gateway events. *Frozen accidents* are best understood as the chance events of the past that have a significant impact on the future. In the shaping of our planet, ecosystem and human evolution, frozen accidents – both big and small – have played an enormous role. Think of the random elements of chance that positioned our planet at an appropriate distance from the life-giving rays of the sun, or the leap from single-celled creatures to multi-celled ones during the early phases of life on Earth. More dramatically, think of the mass extinctions that occurred at the end of the Permian period, 245 million years ago, when more than half of all species on earth disappeared, and during the Cretaceous extinction, about 185 million years later when, due to a massive asteroid strike, dinosaurs became extinct along with one-third of the world's animal and plant life. Without this accident that was frozen into time, the lowly mammals (small furry creatures living in holes in the ground, too insignificant to be of interest to most of the dinosaurs) would have been unable to benefit from the new conditions, and human life as we know it may not have come about.

It is important to note that not all frozen accidents are large ones, like a massive meteorite striking the earth. From a complexity perspective, small changes can also lead to big effects, the so-called 'butterfly effect' that we discussed in Chapter 2. Imagine the relatively miniscule genetic differences between *Homo sapiens* and Neanderthals. Virtually the same basic structure, yet minor differences were enough to tip one species towards extinction and the other towards global domination.

Frozen accidents abound in our daily lives. The chance meeting that leads to a new life course, or the unfortunate event that marks a human tragedy. In many ways, diabetes is a similar frozen accident. Whether it is type 1 or type 2 diabetes, chance played a role in its diagnosis. However, once the 'accident' has occurred and the condition is established, its impact is frozen into the future of that person's life. This doesn't mean that every chance event counts. We are constantly bombarded by chance events and encounters that we ignore, adapt to or overcome, that don't have a major impact on our lives. Just think of the last time you missed a meal. Did this cause you to starve or fall ill? In the vast majority of cases it didn't. However, for a person with diabetes it may be a missed meal that tips them into a hypoglycaemic state. Combine this with a difficult situation – for example, driving late at night – and you have the recipe for a major life catastrophe.

Regularities

Over time, as frozen accidents accumulate, general *regularities* begin to occur that set the boundaries for future developments. For example, in the aftermath of the Big Bang, multiple frozen accidents led to the regularities that created the Milky Way and our own solar system. In the case of human affairs, think of all of the frozen accidents – chance meetings, lucky breaks, geographical features, etc. – that led to the current boundaries of any major city. As cities grow, they establish regularities, such as major travel routes, core industries, and wealthy and poor areas. Regularities may change over time, but they tend to be the more stable aspects of any given complex system or situation. The condition of diabetes is defined by its regularities. Loss of stable blood glucose levels is a form of regularity. Managing diabetes is also very similar. Over time, every person with diabetes evolves regularities – one could call them basic tactics or strategies – for managing their condition. We all follow basic regularities in our daily lives – for example, breathing, eating, and avoiding dangerous situations. The only difference for a person newly diagnosed with diabetes is that they are confronted with adapting to a new set of regularities, and new types of frozen accidents, in a relatively short space of time.

Gateway events

Finally, *gateway events* are in a sense the same as frozen accidents – just seen from the other side. Gateway events are those that open up a whole new range of unpredictable possibilities for complex systems. The first stirrings of life on Earth were a major gateway event for the future of our planet. All the potential for later life was based on that initial event. In human affairs, the creation of language, money or the Internet can be seen as gateway events that significantly broadened the potential variety of human interaction and society. In our individual lives we all experience gateway events – for example, learning a new language, starting a new career or business, getting married, having children – which can all open up huge unknown possibilities in our lives. Gateway events can be both positive and negative. Winning the lottery may be an apparently marvellous gateway event in one's life. However, if it leads the winner to leave his family, quit his job and become addicted to drugs and/or alcohol, then the gateway is more of a trap.

Diabetes is a gateway event for anyone who develops it. It combines new regularities (monitoring diet, exercise, blood glucose levels, etc.) with new unpredictable frozen accidents (integrating one's lifestyle with the new regularities, personal reactions, patient–carer relationship, family response, etc.) in an uneven or punctuated equilibrium way. Once someone passes through the gateway, they can't go back. And that is a very frightening thought. But is it really so different from other gateways that we have all passed through in our lives, such as childhood, puberty, accident and illness? In truth, a whole new landscape of experiences lies in front of that person, some good and some bad. Making the most of the walk through that landscape is what it is really all about. Helping someone to make the most of their walk is what true caring from health professionals and others is all about.

Creating a complexity cascade

Now that we have the concepts, we can bring them all together in one image that captures the evolving nature of complexity, its evolving limits and emergent potentialities. We call this the *cascade of complexity*.[3] It is like a series of fountains stacked on top of each other. The base of each fountain represents a fundamental gateway event that opens the system up to a whole new range of possibilities. Frozen accidents occur that shape the path of the system through the range of possible pathways. Meanwhile, the boundaries of the fountain represent the regularities that emerge that put limits on the possible outcomes. Over time, a new gateway event occurs and a new variety of pathways emerge. The uneven flow of the cascade captures the erratic nature of its punctuated equilibrium. This isn't the smooth and stately progress of a calm stream, but the jerky explosions of stacked fountains.

It applies equally to the physical, biological and human worlds because, from a complexity perspective, human beings are neither a cog in a massive universal machine, nor the pinnacle of universal development. Instead, human beings are complex systems evolving within a larger biological system, within a larger physical one. What does this look like in a complexity cascade?

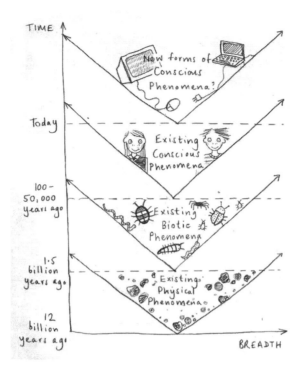

As the picture shows, following the arrow of time and beginning with the Big Bang 12 billion years ago, fundamental physical regularities were created which set the boundaries of existing physical phenomena. These boundaries are extremely wide, but they are still boundaries. Basic physical laws, like gravity, limit the range of physical phenomena. For example, there are no planets right next to each other in the universe. Get close enough and gravity forces them to crash together. They are physically impossible given the basic laws of gravity. Likewise, during the amazing gateway event of the beginnings of life on Earth around 2 billion years ago, the boundaries were set for the evolution of life. As we are well aware, these boundaries are very broad, allowing for bacteria, dinosaurs, fish, humans, etc. However, they do exist. At the very minimum, life as we know it requires certain chemical and physical basics such as oxygen, water and food. Similarly, through the multitude of frozen accidents that led to the emergence of our early human ancestors about 1.8 million years ago, and consciousness, represented by the creation of language in the last 10–50,000 years,[4] the boundaries of existing consciousness were set. Again, other types of consciousness were possible. For example, if the Neanderthals had survived, what form of consciousness and expression would they have evolved? Pushing our imagination further, what kind of imagination would a dolphin have evolved if it had been first on the evolutionary ladder of conscious complexity? Lastly, coming to the present period, we have left open the possibility of new types of consciousness. With the growth of computer power and artificial intelligence, who knows what new type of mixed human/machine consciousness may emerge.[5] The possibilities are both frightening and staggering. Just think of such characters as HAL in the film *2001: A Space Odyssey*, the cyborg machines in *The Terminator,* or the human-like servants in Steven Spielberg's *A.I.*

Diabetes and the complexity cascade

Coming back down to the here and now, how does all of this relate to diabetes? Similar to our complexity mapping boxes in Chapter 3, this massively broad image provides an excellent metaphor for understanding diabetes and its effects on patients, carers and health professionals.

Let us start with an imaginary patient, Mark, a 72-year-old retired fireman. He started working as a fireman when he was 20, and got married in the same year. His life went well, with no major health difficulties, a stable family life and three healthy children. He retired at 58 and his wife died of breast cancer when he was 62. Despite having good relationships with his children and grandchildren, he began to feel more and more depressed and isolated. He was less active and put on weight. At the age of 68 he was diagnosed with type 2 diabetes.

If we stop here and look at Mark's life, we can see how it exhibits all of the main complexity concepts that we have talked about in this chapter. Starting with the frozen accident of his birth – accidental in the sense of which sperm hitting which egg, and frozen in that once this mixture is in place his basic genetic makeup is now set – Mark's life goes through a series of major gateway events (marriage, career, retirement, etc.) that open up a range of possible new experiences. As choices are made, regularities emerge. His genetic code is set at birth – for example, he can't be a genetic female. He stays married and faithful to his wife, thereby limiting his sexual partners. He remains a fireman, limiting his experience of other jobs, but overall his life exhibits all of the main aspects of change and stability that typify punctuated equilibrium. In a general sense his personal complexity cascade would look like Figure 6.1.

Now if we look at Mark's life since he received the bad news that he had diabetes, a similar complexity cascade emerges. Again, the frozen accident of diabetes added a new layer of boundaries, possibilities and challenges in his life. At first he dealt with it poorly, feeling more isolated and taking no exercise. He understood the need to control his diet and be more active, but he just couldn't get motivated. He was slowly building in negative regularities into his life (poor diet, no exercise, and depression). His children were busy with their own lives and didn't seem really able to help. His doctor was informative but very busy as well. After several discussions, the doctor mentioned a new health club that was opening up near where Mark lived. Mark had no intention of going, but saw an advert in the paper that said 'One week for free for new members.' He thought 'Why not?' He met Joan on the first day. She was the receptionist at the club, had a wonderful smile and Mark was smitten. On their first 'date', Mark found out that Joan had diabetes as well. All of a sudden, Mark had someone to share his diabetes with. Going to the club to see Joan became a daily routine. His weight, diet and blood glucose control all began to improve. He was now building in positive regularities that made it easier and easier to deal with his diabetes. A whole new way of living seemed to open up to him. Building on the previous figure, Mark's diabetes complexity cascade would now look something like Figure 6.2.

Where did it all begin? With his meeting Joan, with his doctor, with his getting diabetes, or with his knowledge of the joys, strengths and weaknesses of having a life

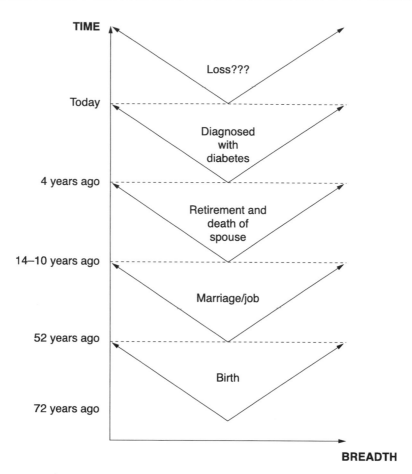

Figure 6.1: Mark's complexity cascade.

partner that he learned about when he was living with his first wife? There is no simple answer! The key point from a complexity perspective is that the cascade of complexity never stops until we are dead. That is when we truly become the orderly actors that the mechanistic perspective always wanted us to be. And even then, in many ways our personal cascades live on in the memories, thoughts and actions of those whose lives we have touched.

Do you need to have diabetes to have a complexity cascade?

What about the other people in Mark's life, his doctor and family members? Can we view Mark's diabetes through their complexity cascades?

Let's imagine Emily, Mark's GP. She is 45 and living with a male partner. She likes being a GP but is uncertain whether she needs something more in her life. She had a good but traditional medical training that set the general boundaries of her approach to health and medicine. The numerous NHS reorganisations and increased pressures

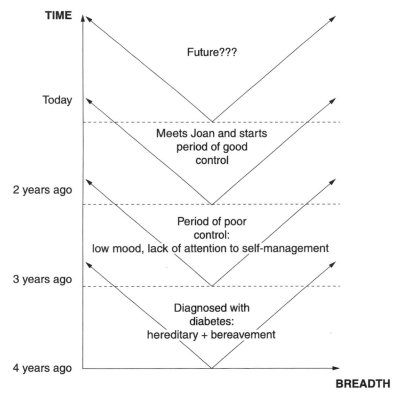

Figure 6.2: Mark's diabetes complexity cascade.

for GP efficiency have pushed her to become even more 'orderly' in her approach to illness and her patients. She is up to date on diabetes and has read about more holistic and complementary approaches, but has no time to actually apply them. To get through her day she allocates 6 minutes per patient. She has a few people with type 1 diabetes, but a much larger number of type 2 patients.

She met Mark 4 years ago. She liked him straight away. Her father had been a fireman as well. In Emily's eyes, Mark was a typical type 2 patient – elderly, low activity levels with mild symptoms. He was easily dealt with within the 6-minute time slot. However, instead of improving he seemed to do poorly from the start. Two years later, after multiple visits and clear evidence of inadequate control, Emily couldn't think of anything other than to repeat the basics – good diet, exercise, altered drug treatment and screen for complications. In mild exasperation at the end of one 6-minute session she suggested a new health club for Mark. She had forgotten about it by the time the next patient opened her door.

It was some time before she saw Mark again. He had come in about his vision. It was fine but he might eventually need a simple cataract operation. She was stunned at how well he looked. He had clearly lost weight and gained fitness. 'It was your suggestion about the health club that did it', said Mark. 'This may sound strange, but going there was one of the best decisions of my life.' Emily was stunned. She had been telling him to exercise from the beginning. Why had it worked now? After a little questioning, Mark eventually mentioned Joan and how she had made him rethink diabetes and his

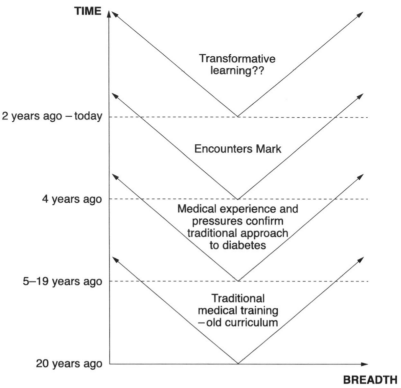

Figure 6.3: Emily's complexity cascade.

own life. When Mark left, Emily had to reflect on what Mark had said. Something so small had made a huge difference in his life. What had this taught her? Like Mark, Emily was on the brink of a gateway event, particularly in relation to understanding that traditional approaches to management are limited when dealing with chronic diseases such as diabetes.

Janet is Mark's daughter. She is 48, divorced, manages a flower shop and has three children (aged 24, 21 and 18). She has a very busy life. As the children have started leaving home, Janet's job has taken up more and more of her time. She has always had a reasonably good relationship with her father. However, she was much closer to her mother, so her death left her feeling bereft. When her father was also diagnosed with diabetes her first feelings were ones of fear – fear for her father and fear of having to take care of him. She was finally getting the kids out of the house. The last thing she wanted was the added pressure of caring for an ill parent! Also, what about the financial burden? Mark had a pension, but would that be enough if things got really difficult?

Janet read the handouts on diabetes and listened carefully to the doctor. At first she was relieved. 'It wasn't so bad after all', she thought. 'If he takes care of himself it shouldn't be any problem.' Unfortunately, things went badly right from the start. Her father wasn't taking care of himself. Janet's fears grew and she started to pressure her father to do *exactly* what the doctors said. Not surprisingly, this backfired and Mark stopped seeing Janet as often as he had been doing, and started to hide his problems.

Janet felt guilty and responded by working longer and harder at the flower shop. Weeks would go by and she wouldn't hear from her father. When they did talk she knew things were going wrong, but did her best to ignore them.

The first hint of a change was when Janet's friend, Ross, told her that he had seen her father at the fitness club. She made a mental note to call him about this, but forgot. Six weeks later, Mark called her and invited her out for dinner. They hadn't gone out for dinner since before he was diagnosed with diabetes. When she saw him she was stunned at the change in him. He had lost some weight and seemed to have some of his old energy back. Equally startling, he had a new female friend. Although she was unsure at first, Janet realised where the real difficulty lay. The death of her mother had hit Mark hard. He was lonely and afraid. The diabetes had merely amplified these feelings. He felt he couldn't cope and wasn't even sure if he wanted to. Joan had given him something to live for. Maybe this was even a lesson for herself – that there might be other aspects to life than working in the flower shop. Like her father, Janet was on her own complexity cascade, learning that changes in life – good and bad – contribute towards its ever changing variety. How we walk through our experiences and what we learn and make from them is the real value of who we are.

For Janet, her complexity cascade during her father's experience with diabetes would look something like the following.

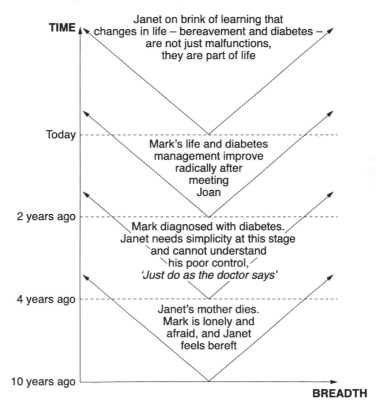

Figure 6.4: Janet's complexity cascade.

The cascade of complexity game

Just as we did in Chapter 2 with the boxes, you can make your own complexity cascade for your own life and your experience with diabetes. Ask yourself what have been the main gateway events and regularities (both positive and negative) that have played a major role in your life. Then make a complexity cascade of your life. How has your life changed? Has it really changed at all? Get others to do this exercise as well. Again, there are no right or wrong answers, just a way of perceiving the signposts on your journey through your own complexity cascade.

References

1 Gould S. *The Mismeasure of Man.* New York: WW Norton; 1996.
2 Coveney P, Highfield R. *Frontiers of Complexity: the search for order in a chaotic world.* London: Faber and Faber; 1995.
3 Geyer R. *Is There Anything to Fear From the Politics of Complexity?* Presentation to London School of Economics Complexity Group; www.psych.lse.ac.uk/complexity/index.html (accessed 1 July 2006).
4 Morowitz H. *The Emergence of Everything: how the world became complex.* Oxford: Oxford University Press; 2002. p. 156.
5 Mainzer K. *Thinking in Complexity: the computational dynamics of matter, mind, and mankind.* Berlin: Springer; 2004.

Further reading on these complexity concepts

Briggs J, Peat FD. *Turbulent Mirror: an illustrated guide to chaos theory and the science of wholeness.* New York: Harper and Row; 1989.
Byrne D. *Complexity Theory and the Social Sciences.* London: Routledge; 1998.
Coveney P, Highfield R. *Frontiers of Complexity: the search for order in a chaotic world.* London: Faber and Faber; 1995.
Geyer R, Mackintosh A. *Integrating UK and European Social Policy: the complexity of Europeanisation.* Oxford: Radcliffe Publishing; 2005.
Lewin R. *Complexity: life at the edge of chaos.* Chicago: University of Chicago Press; 1992.
Waldrop M. *Complexity: the emerging science at the edge of order and chaos.* New York: Simon and Schuster; 1992.

Chapter 7

Complementary management of diabetes

Evolution is a tightly coupled dance, with life and the material environment as partners. From the dance emerges the entity Gaia.
(Interview with James Lovelock, author of the ground-breaking and controversial *Gaia: A New Look at Life on Earth*)

People see life through a cultural filter.
(Laurence Evans, *Nature's Holism: Holism, Ecology and Evolution*)

James Lovelock is a feisty and fascinating character. Born in Letchworth Garden City, UK in 1919, he obtained a PhD in Medicine from the London School of Hygiene and Tropical Medicine in 1949, but his real passion was inventing. While working for a number of universities he filed over 50 patents for inventions, mostly for use in chemical detection in the environment. In the 1960s, while he was working for NASA on detectors to determine whether there was life on Mars, he was struck by the difference between the stability of the lifelessness on Mars and the continually evolving physical, chemical and biological changes on our life-giving Earth. In essence, for Lovelock the Earth is not just a ball of rock with life on top, but a kind of super-organism composed of interwoven physical, chemical and biological systems. He called this super-organism *Gaia* (the name of the Greek goddess of the Earth).

When his first major book was published in 1979, he was generally shunned by the scientific community, as his ideas flew in the face of their traditional thinking that wanted to keep the different elements of life (biological, physical, psychological and social) in simplistic isolated boxes. Over time, with the growth of the environmental movement and the growing recognition of the impact of global warming, Lovelock's ideas have helped to reshape environmental studies and national and international policies. But what does this have to do with diabetes?

Well, it links with it in two ways. First, diabetes emerges as a result of a breakdown in the body's carbohydrate self-regulating mechanism. This impacts upon other systems in the body, and if not controlled it results over time in complications mediated through effects on the vascular and nervous systems. In other words, like Gaia theory, diabetes is best understood as a web of systems and/or activities that interrelate so that a breakdown in one affects others. What this indicates is that if we want to truly understand diabetes – and ultimately manage the disease – then we must think about networks. This, like Gaia, has practical implications. If we treat the system badly, then the self-regulatory mechanisms stop working effectively and the body can no longer heal itself. In this sense, environmental pollution and the associated explosion of greenhouse gases and subsequent global warming have clear parallels with the obesity crisis affecting the world's wealthiest countries and the subsequent rise of diabetes. In both cases 'An ounce of prevention is worth a pound of cure'!

Secondly, Lovelock's idea that we are intertwined with our environment means that we develop ideas that reflect common thinking within that place and time. As our second opening quote emphasises, we are always 'biased' in our thinking, particularly in the way in which we view health and illness and their management. As we saw in earlier chapters, with the arrogance of scientific certainty we have adopted the so-called Western or orthodox philosophy of medicine with its focus on 'control' – typified by its rigorous training and registration of practitioners, its reliance upon drugs, and its progressive search for treatments that are sustained by a 'hard' evidence base. However, modern medicine has only truly been around for about 100 years, compared with, say, Chinese medicinal herbs and acupressure, which have been around since the *I Ching* (also known as the *Book of Changes)* was written over 4000 years ago. It is now generally acknowledged that only a fraction of our increased longevity is a result of modern medicine. The rest can be attributed quite simply to improved living conditions associated with better sanitation and nutrition, and reductions in childhood infections.[1] Alongside this, we now have a growing epidemic of illnesses (some forms of diabetes among them) that are resulting from our unhealthy lifestyles and which traditional approaches to medicine are finding difficult to 'control' – for example, overeating, lack of exercise, stress, alcohol consumption and, of course, smoking. Given this, it is important to acknowledge both the value of modern medicine and its shortcomings.

Alternatives to the dominant modern approach

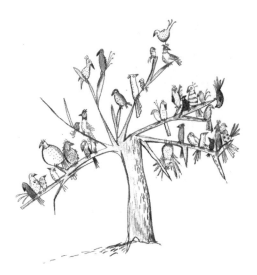

There is a Burmese saying, 'Ten thousand birds can perch on one good tree' that reflects our dependence in the Western world on modern medicine, a dependence created by the aura of its protective strength. However, the strength of this 'tree' is beginning to be challenged as we confront new problems. Lifestyle-related diseases, a growing elderly population with associated rises in chronic diseases, increasing prevalence of cancers, old infectious diseases showing their faces again (e.g. TB)

alongside relatively new types of infectious diseases (e.g. HIV/AIDS), and antibiotic-resistant infections (e.g. MRSA) are increasingly challenging modern medicine. Finding a way through these problems has led people to search for other forms of therapy to enhance our accepted Western traditions. This search has raised the profile of complementary therapies so that the line between modern and complementary medicine is now becoming blurred.

For most of us in the UK, complementary therapy has played a marginal role, but it constitutes mainstream thinking in other cultures. It covers lifestyle therapies such as meditation and relaxation, Eastern therapies such as Chinese medicine and acupuncture, natural theories such as herbalism and homeopathy, manipulative therapies such as chiropractice and osteopathy, mind therapies such as hypnotherapy and spiritual healing, and art therapies such as dance, music and art. Under modern medicine there is a clear separation between mind and body that goes all the way back to the French philosopher, Descartes, who regarded the body as a clockwork mechanism.[2] Complementary therapies, like complexity theory, do not accept this separation, and they focus on the interrelationships between the mind and body. Modern medicine, with its focus on managing the physicality of disease by using drugs (a position heartily supported by a massive global pharmaceutical industry), has tended to isolate the body from the mind. Combining modern and complementary medicine should be able to make the best of both approaches and would seem to be common sense. However, the 'scientific' barrier that lies between them is both a lack of research to prove the effectiveness of complementary therapies, and the difficulties in applying the methods of conventional medical research to such treatments. But let us look more closely at how they fit together for diabetes, using complexity to guide our arguments.

Learning to think 'complementarily'

If we go back to Chapter 5, with its focus on the way things interconnect and the need for an inclusive management model, then we have a place within complexity for the idea of blurring the boundaries between traditional and complementary therapies. In that chapter, we located complexity in Stacey's zone 5, where traditional 'command-and-control' management approaches tend not to 'fit.' This is the area where people need to learn new approaches and new techniques, and maybe even unlearn tried and tested methods. It is the region where we experiment and learn through trial and error. So let us consider the process of *learning* in more detail.

Learning about diabetes – be it as a practitioner, a patient or a carer – is an experiential process. As such it includes three simultaneous and integrated dimensions, namely a cognitive or knowledge dimension, an emotional, attitudinal and motivational or psychological dimension, and a social dimension. Each of these dimensions occurs in two processes which, although different, are always integrated, namely the internal acquisition process and the external interaction process between the learner and the material and social environment. Much of our learning about diabetes therefore takes time – it emerges through the process of living and working with the disease. Given this, there is a need to acknowledge that emergence of such learning requires the following:

- self-organisation

- the ability to be able to deal with new problems as they arise
- the ability to connect things together to make sense of what is happening
- recognition of the fact that perfection is not always possible, so mistakes will happen
- acceptance that life with diabetes can at times seem chaotic.

These ideas have much in common with a complexity perspective which, as our boxes have illustrated, is composed of orderly, complex and disorderly elements. To ignore this complexity is to fundamentally reject the basic reality that surrounds us when we are trying to deal with diabetes.

If we take these ideas to explore 'treatment' in all of its forms, we need to acknowledge that management of diabetes, interwoven as it is within the context of an individual's life, involves processes that are too varied for us to understand in simple mechanistic ways. As we know, not all factors can be controlled completely through the use of drugs, diet and exercise. For some, complementary therapies fill a gap. Complexity therefore provides a structure which allows for both traditional and complementary therapies. If you will, traditional interventions are for the orderly bits and complementary strategies for the more complex bits. Not surprisingly, this can be visualised with the following (which is similar to Figure 3.5 in Chapter 3):

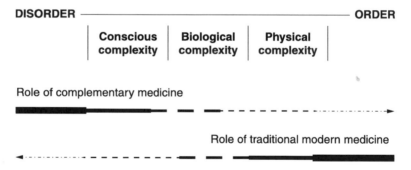

Figure 7.1 Decision making in a complexity perspective.

But how can we prove that complementary strategies work when they are on the more uncertain, complexity and disorderly side of our scale? To answer this question, instead of reviewing the wide range of complementary therapies for which there is little if any clinical evidence to support their use in diabetes, we shall focus on 'relaxation therapy' which is now widely accepted.

Relaxation therapy and diabetes: exploring the evidence

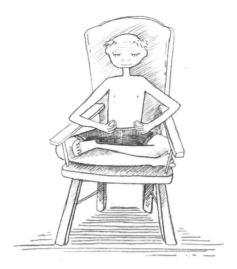

As everyone knows, stress is all around us and is a central part of our lives. In our pre-modern times, when our noses picked up a strange scent or we heard a threatening sound, our autonomic nervous system released adrenaline into our bodies to prepare us to fight or flee. Our heart and breathing rates soared, our muscles tightened and our pupils dilated in preparation for the threat or opportunity. This is an excellent system, and it was central to human survival for millions of years. However, in the space of a few thousand years humans have radically transformed their local environment into a much less threatening and more inactive one. At the same time, there has been a great increase in social and personal 'stressors' – the consequence of living in larger and larger groups. The result is that overall stress has increased, alongside changes in nutrition and a reduction in physical activity, both of which can help to alleviate the body's responses to stress. As usual, with diabetes the situation is even more complicated.

For people with diabetes, stress induces a number of complicating reactions, including the following:

- inhibition of pancreatic insulin secretion, where insulin is still being produced, as in type 2 diabetes
- inhibition of glucose uptake from the blood and oxidation by many body cells – so-called 'insulin antagonism'
- stimulation of gluconeogenesis (i.e. the production of glucose from glycogen stores in the liver and from sources other than carbohydrates).

All of these reactions can raise blood glucose levels directly. Stress-induced hormones also increase blood pressure, worsen insulin resistance and stimulate hyperlipidaemia (high cholesterol levels) through lipolysis (breakdown of fats with a resultant increase in circulating free fatty acids). Such an energy mobilisation response (useful though it was to outrun a hungry bear) is potentially harmful in people who have diabetes, given the relative or absolute deficiency of insulin, hyperglycaemia, hyperlipidaemia and/or insulin resistance that characterise the illness. Stress can also impact on glucose control indirectly through the effect of individual behaviours – for example, 'comfort' eating or drinking alcohol in order to 'feel better.' Given these interconnected effects, it seems startling to realise that stress management techniques have never been a central part of mainstream diabetes management programmes! The obvious question is 'Why not?'

The answer to this conundrum lies within the limited focus of 'mechanical' Western medicine and its continued mind–body separation. For example, relaxation is something that we all do and is obviously very important to our lives. Yet for people under stress, a state of relaxation can seem impossible to achieve. Unfortunately, because modern medicine views diabetes as a predominantly physical problem, the psychological implications – the mind games – are often downplayed, ignored, or approached through a primarily body-oriented lens, with drugs being offered as the solution. From this perspective the physical interventions can solve the problem and there is no need for or inherent benefit to the patient of learning relaxation techniques. It is much easier (particularly for the health professional, who can write out a quick prescription and go on to the next patient) to take a pill. It is only very recently that non-pill-based approaches, such as cognitive behavioural therapy, have begun to achieve widespread recognition.

In addition to this 'pill-popping' bias, modern medical research with its mechanical orientation has generally ignored the vague and fuzzy areas of complementary medicine such as relaxation therapy. In fact, it is only in the last 10 to 20 years that major research has begun to explore the impact and potential benefits of relaxation therapies. Early studies were not promising. For example, a systematic review of research studies concerning education and psychosocial interventions for people with diabetes found that relaxation training did not have a major impact on blood glucose control.[3] Another extensive evaluation of relaxation training in people who had type 2 diabetes reinforced these results.[4] In this later study, 38 randomly selected individuals (a very, very small number of people!) were given conventional intensive diabetes therapy, with half (19 individuals) also having eight weekly sessions of relaxation training (a very short course of relaxation training!). Blood glucose control improved in both groups, but with no extra benefit for the group that received the relaxation training. However, and this is the important point, the researchers found that even given this very short relaxation course, for the more anxious patients the relaxation training selectively helped them to feel much better about their condition, potentially leading to better management in the long term. This conclusion was reinforced later by Aikens et al.[5]

In another study, Hendricks and Hendricks[6] investigated patients' feelings about having type 2 diabetes, and found that they had major fears about the long-term complications associated with the disease. These researchers concluded that an important step in improving patient welfare would be to help patients to deal with these fears. Zettler et al.,[7] using a group therapy programme (which included relaxation training and analysis of dysfunctional health beliefs) for people with diabetes, found that the therapy significantly improved the patients' ability to cope with the fear of long-term complications. They found significant improvements with regard to fear and acceptance of diabetes, despite the fact that there were no significant short-term changes in blood glucose levels. The authors concluded that this type of therapy provided support for patients in dealing with the issues surrounding the fears of long-term complications of diabetes. In essence, relaxation therapy alongside psychological support appeared to help the patients to gain a sense of 'wellness' that simple pill-based interventions could not offer.

So what does all of this tell us? The emerging research suggests that relaxation may have a beneficial effect on how people cope with the psychological effects of having diabetes – mind games, as we know, being an integral part of the diabetes experiential learning process. Thus there is not so much a lack of evidence with regard to complementary therapies, as a lack of the right type of evidence. In other words, the evidence accumulated so far is limited because of its focus on the researcher's (and practitioner's) traditional biomedical measurement of blood glucose control and, important as this is to everyone, it totally underestimates the importance of emotional factors (the sense of 'wellness') that contribute to the experience of living and coping with diabetes. Patients, on the other hand, may feel that a sense of 'wellness' is just as important as or even more important than blood glucose control. For as complexity and common sense tell us, we are more than the sum of our parts, and diabetes is more than mere blood glucose control. Just read through the poem below, written by a 13-year-old person living with diabetes, describing what it feels like to have a hypo. No amount of measurement of blood glucose levels could capture what he has written here:

I Wait

I'm having a hypo
And although I know
I wait.
I hope I'm imagining it
I wait some more
Just a bit
Oh no, it is a hypo
I'll have to change my insulin again
What a pain
That's four times this week.
At half past
I drop my pen
And reach for the glucose in my pocket.
It's really hard to move my arm
As if it's slipped out of its socket.
My body feels drained
Of all its blood
My legs feel like dead slabs of wood
I'm feeling shattered
I start to sweat
I swallow another glucose tablet
I wait.
Some time later I am well
But at the time it was hell.[8]

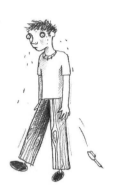

And the world beyond relaxation: Chinese medicine, placebo effects, acupuncture, herbal therapies . . .

Relaxation therapy is just the beginning. A whole range of complementary approaches are just beginning to be explored or are just emerging, which we can only touch upon in this book. An interesting area of research is the use of traditional Chinese herbal medicines. In a systematic review of research trials, these were found to have some hypoglycaemic effects in type 2 diabetes, and further high-quality trials are planned.[9] Another systematic review of the published literature on the efficacy and safety of herbal therapies and vitamin/mineral supplements for glucose control in patients with diabetes concluded that several supplements warrant further study.[10]

Another area that deserves mention is the 'placebo effect.' From the Western angle, the placebo effect is felt to exert itself in some mysterious way. It is defined as a measurable, observable or felt improvement in health that is not attributable to treatment. A prime example is the effect of faith or spiritual healers. You may have seen the TV programmes where people appear to get up and walk after having been invalided for many years, you may well have been sceptical about the truth of such happenings, and in some cases you should be! However, the placebo effect is not some sideshow. It can be more powerful than drugs or even surgery. In one experiment, people were duped into believing that they had received knee surgery and, incredibly, this so-called 'sham' group of patients did as well as those who had undergone the real procedure.[11] This is not to argue that placebos can effectively treat diabetes, but it does show that a patient's state of mind – their sense of 'wellness' – can have a powerful impact on their actions, their feeling for their condition, and even to some extent the outcome of that condition.

Two final areas to mention are acupuncture and herbal remedies. Again, ancient Chinese health practices have been shown to have significant impacts on the mental and physical well-being of patients. For example, by examining brain scans that show states of pain, researchers found that acupuncture stimulates chemical changes in the body, mediated through the limbic system in the brain, that can have a major impact on pain and the sensation of pain.[12] And then there is herbalism. Research in its early stages has suggested that certain plants, such as garlic, contain much more than a couple of active ingredients. They are enormously complex chemical cocktails with medicinal properties that modern pharmaceuticals simply can't reproduce.[13] Researchers are only just beginning to explore how diets with a high content of complex herbs, such as garlic, may impact on the chronic disease experience.

What all this emerging evidence tells us is that traditional Western medicine is beginning to acknowledge a place for complementary therapies, and in doing so, is starting to acknowledge that new research philosophies are required to enhance the current methodologies. Proven efficacy, although essential, needs to be expanded to include other variables that are just as important to those who live and work with diseases such as diabetes. So while Western-style medicine focuses on physical (external) effects and complementary therapies look inside, the patient and practitioner may need to combine the two approaches in their own unique way. Complementary therapies may therefore be useful as an adjunct treatment, or may be included in a comprehensive management programme. Complexity provides a theoretical framework for such adjustments, and as evidence of effectiveness accumulates, a marriage of traditional and complementary therapies will allow a variety of treatments to flourish in happy coexistence. From any perspective, unity in diversity seems to be the principle for managing diabetes. Following the argument of the punctuated equilibrium, there is no final stable equilibrium for treatment. It needs to evolve, and for us here in the West, orthodox medicine has been just part of that journey.

What can you do now?

Whether you are a patient, a carer, a practitioner or a researcher, why not try a relaxation therapy for yourself? There is a whole range of books and Internet resources to choose from. In addition to these, relaxation and meditation tapes are readily available in most major book and music shops. Moreover, if you are a patient, carer or doctor, don't be afraid to share your relaxation strategies with others. The most powerful learning comes through sharing your experience with others.

Have a go

Below are descriptions of three simple relaxation techniques that are among our personal favourites. They are not new or radical in any sense. Again, this is not just for patients! If you are a carer or practitioner you should also try them, and not only for your own well-being. For how can you expect to fully explain the techniques to someone else if you haven't tried them yourself? Hopefully if you try them you may start to get something of a feel for what these strategies can do. It is just a little step down a very long road, but as the butterfly effect shows, small changes can have big effects – and it may even prove to be a 'gateway event' in your life!

A calm word

This technique is inspired by Paul Wilson's *Big Book of Calm*, and is merely the simple repetition of a calming word. It can be used anywhere and at any time, but is most effective if practised in a quiet place for 10–15 minutes at a time. If possible, sit or lie down in a relaxed position with your back straight, your arms and legs unfolded and all tight clothing loosened or removed. Close your eyes and focus your mind on taking deep slow breaths. As you exhale, very softly repeat your calm word. The choice of your calming word is really up to you, but should be short, simple and relaxing. Any of the following words will do:

- calm
- stillness
- harmony
- tranquil
- content
- peace
- serene.

For those who are unfamiliar with relaxation techniques, this may seem absurdly simplistic. Yet it is one of the most effective, and can be surprisingly difficult. For as you are repeating your word your mind will very naturally jump from one thing to another – the day's events, a past crisis, a future fear. Sometimes it will constantly return to an aspect of your life, particularly a fear of future events.

Why does the mind do this? An excellent analogy for the way the mind focuses on some fears is the method that local hunters in parts of Asia use to catch monkeys. The hunter takes a coconut, cuts a small hole in it, inserts a banana and leaves it for the monkey to find. When the monkey finds the coconut, it grabs the banana but can't get it out of the hole and is unwilling to let go. Burdened by the weight of the coconut, the monkey cannot climb a tree and is easily captured by the hunter. Like the monkey, our minds will occasionally focus on something and won't let go, even if we know that the fear is unjustified and that the constant focusing is making us anxious and unwell. The difference is that we can teach ourselves to let go, but this takes time and practice.

While you are practising your relaxation exercises and your mind is jumping about or focusing on one fear, as it surely will, return your mind to your calming word. Try not to force your mind back to your word, but try to let your fear go and then return to your word. In the beginning this will be very difficult, but with time and practice it will become easier. If possible, try to make time for at least one calm session per day.

What is the science behind repeated self-suggestion? Stacks of books in the fields of psychotherapeutic and behaviour therapies have been written on self-suggestion. Basically, it works by helping to break the mind's focus on fears that create a general sense of anxiety. If you can refocus your mind towards calming thoughts, you may be able to learn how to let go of your fears. The key lesson is that you won't solve or conquer them, but you can learn to live with them and realise that they are a normal part of your complex life.

One point to remember is that this technique can be used for much shorter periods and in more chaotic places. For example, one of our favourite places for using this technique is in the car while waiting at a red light. Rather than sitting there gripping the steering wheel ever tighter and wishing the world would go faster, why not take the moment to breathe deeply and slowly and repeat your calm word until the light changes? You will get wherever you are going just as fast, and you will get there in a much healthier frame of mind. Just don't close your eyes!

Training your body to relax

This technique is similar to one described in Stephan Bodian's book *Meditation for Dummies*. As in the previous exercise, find a calm place where you can sit or lie quietly in a relaxed position with your back straight, your arms and legs unfolded and all tight clothing loosened or removed. Close your eyes and focus your mind on taking deep slow breaths. This time, instead of repeating your calming word, focus your attention on relaxing your body. Begin by focusing on your hands. Try to feel the weight of each hand. Feel gravity pulling on it. Focus on that feeling and try to allow your hands to relax. You may even feel the blood pulsing through them. If you like, repeat your calm word as you focus on relaxing your hands. When you hands are relaxed, move to your forearms. Feel their weight. Feel the relaxation of your hands spreading to your arms. Say your calm word if you like. When your forearms are relaxed, move to your upper arms, and then on to your shoulders. Allow the relaxation to move up both arms and connect at the base of your neck. Focus your mind on the core of your body and try to feel the flow of your breath, the beating of your heart and the motion of your belly. These are all wondrous things that we so often ignore. Imagine a feeling of relaxation flowing down to your legs and into your feet. Finally, return to your shoulders and allow the relaxation to flow up your neck and around the back of your head. Imagine a wave of warm relaxation moving slowly from the top of your head to the tip of your nose and down to your chin. Feel your face relaxing, your jaw becoming more slack and your forehead smoothing. When you have finished your tour of your body, allow yourself to enjoy the experience and the feeling of relaxation.

By the way, this is an excellent bedtime routine to help you fall asleep, or for relaxing you if you are lying awake at night!

Ten steps to a relaxed state of mind

This technique is a variation of one described in Jon Kabat-Zinn's excellent book *Full Catastrophe Living*. As above, find a calm place where you can sit or lie quietly in a relaxed position with your back straight, your arms and legs unfolded and all tight clothing loosened or removed. Close your eyes and focus your mind on taking deep slow breaths. This time, instead of repeating your calming word, focus your attention on your hands. Feel them relaxing and getting heavy. Then focus on one finger/thumb on one hand, take a calming breath and quietly say the word 'non-striving.' Focus on the next finger, take a breath, and say 'non-judging.' Repeat this exercise on your remaining fingers/thumb with the following words:

- open mind
- trust
- patience
- acceptance
- letting go
- calm
- tranquil
- content.

Why are these words important? Each word holds an important lesson in learning how to relax.

- *Non-striving* is important because we spend so much of our lives racing after the next deadline, job, relationship, etc. that we often forget what is important and who we are. Meditating on just being, rather than striving for the next goal, is a key step in learning how to relax.
- *Non-judging* is very similar. We are constantly judging situations, people and events, which leads us on an emotional rollercoaster throughout our day. Non-judging is about stepping back from the automatic judging process and accepting the complex, ever-changing world as it is.
- *Open mind* merely encourages you to view every experience and day as if it were a new and special one. Try to peel away the layers of judging and indulge yourself in the sensations of a deep breath, warm toes, the sound of a bird or the thought of a loved one.
- *Trust* is about learning how to trust yourself and your feelings. Fundamentally, relaxation is about being more relaxed with yourself. To do this, you need to trust yourself and your feelings.
- *Patience.* Many events unfold at their own pace – a butterfly from a chrysalis, an adult from childhood. Patience teaches us to accept the world as it is and give it the time to make its own changes.
- *Acceptance,* like patience, encourages us to see the world as it is in the present with all its good and bad aspects. It isn't about being passive, but about truly recognising ourselves and situations. One must first accept, before one can change.
- *Letting go* is a particularly important idea. Again, since much of our time is spent chasing after people, events and situations, meditation and relaxation are about practising 'letting go' of our striving, judging and impatience and accepting the present for what it is.
- The final three words, *calm, tranquil* and *content,* are merely reminders of the importance of relaxation for the creation of a calm, tranquil and content mind and life.

Lastly, after you have gone through your 10 words on your hands, reward yourself with deep breaths and the repetition of the word *peace.* Feel the sense of peace spreading from your hands, up through your arms, into your neck and shoulders and from there throughout your whole body. Repeat the exercise as you like.

References

1 Wilmoth JR. Demography of longevity: past, present and future trends. *Exp Gerontol.* 2000; **35:** 1111–29.
2 Mainzer K. *Thinking in Complexity: the computational dynamics of matter, mind and mankind.* 4th ed. Berlin: Springer; 2004.
3 Padgett D, Mumford E, Hynes M *et al.* Meta-analysis of the effects of educational and psychosocial interventions on management of diabetes mellitus. *J Clin Epidemiol.* 1988; **41:** 1007–30.
4 Lane JD *et al.* Relaxation training for NIDDM. Predicting who may benefit. *Diabetes Care.* 1993; **16:** 1087–94.

5 Aikens JE, Kiolbasa TA, Sobel R. Psychological predictors of glycaemic change with relaxation training in non-insulin-dependent diabetes mellitus. *Psychother Psychosom.* 1997; **66:** 302–6.

6 Hendricks LE, Hendricks RT. Greatest fears of Type 1 and Type 2 patients about having diabetes: implications for diabetes educators. *Diabetes Educ.* 1998; **24:** 168–73.

7 Zettler A, Duran G, Waadt S *et al.* Coping with fear of complications in diabetes mellitus: a model clinical program. *Psychother Psychosom.* 1995; **64:** 178–84.

8 Cooper H, Williams G, editors. *A Collection of Poems Written by Children With Diabetes and Their Parents, in Aid of Liverpool Diabetes Research Action Fund.* Supported by a grant from Eli Lilly and Company Ltd. Unpublished; 1998.

9 Liu JP, Zhang M, Wang WY *et al.* Chinese herbal medicines for type 2 diabetes mellitus. In: *The Cochrane Database of Systematic Reviews. Issue 3.* Oxford: Update Software; 2002.

10 Yeh G, Eisenberg DM, Kaptchuk TJ *et al.* Systematic review of herbs and dietary supplements for glycemic control in diabetes. *Diabetes Care.* 2003; **26:** 1277–94.

11 Moseley JB, O'Malley K, Petersen NJ *et al.* A controlled trial of arthroscopic surgery for osteoarthritis of the knee. *NEJM.* 2002; **347:** 81–8.

12 Hui KKS, Liu J, Makris N *et al.* Acupuncture modulates the limbic system and subcortical gray structures of the human brain: evidence from studies in normal subjects. *Hum Brain Mapping.* 2000; **9:** 13–25.

13 www.open2.net/alternativemedicine/index.html (accessed July 2006).

Chapter 8

A call for personal and professional reaction

> You gotta go there to come back.
> (Recent hit CD by the Stereophonics)

To bring this book to a close we want to highlight a number of what we feel are the most important key general lessons to take from complexity thinking. But before we do this, have a go for yourself. What things do you remember? What has stayed with you? Write a list and then see how it compares with our 'take-home' messages. Don't think too hard about it – just write down what comes into your head.

Getting a good 'balance' and taking responsibility for your own 'balance'

As the tools of complexity hopefully make clear, managing complex systems and phenomena such as diabetes is more complicated than merely repeating a few simple rules. Yes, there are always core rules to follow – don't smoke, eat a reasonable diet, take regular exercise, etc. – but beyond that everything quickly gets fuzzy. For example, what are the best tactics to follow in order to stop smoking, eat a reasonable diet and take regular exercise? Health professionals, carers and friends can help with advice, suggestions, recommendations and so on, but in the end the key is to encourage patients to find their own balance, or as the medical literature says, for patients to become good 'self-managers.' The role of the professional and the carer then becomes one of 'mentor' rather than 'teacher.'

The problem with this seemingly common-sense position is that it flies in the face of centuries of traditional thinking. If there is underlying order, then experts with greater knowledge and skills are obviously best placed to advise a patient on what to do. In this scenario, patients are passive actors who feel obliged to do as they are told – reminiscent of the school environment! Meanwhile, carers are the enforcers in the system, making sure that patients don't cheat. As we have tried to show, from a complexity perspective not only are we all 'experts' in our own areas, but we are all exploring and learning as we go along. In essence, patients, carers and health professionals are therefore all making their own balances in managing diabetes. Health professionals are busy weighing up possible evidence and similarities with other cases to try to give the best advice for a particular patient – not an easy thing to do in a money- and time-pressured environment where getting to know the patient is often seen as a luxury. Carers struggle to match the needs of the patient to the medical advice. Patients can sometimes feel caught in a frightening and difficult situation that can seem foreign and out of control.

No wonder that we all want to revert to the traditional thinking – after all it is a well-trodden path. The doctor should know what to do, and any failures can then be 'blamed' on patient weaknesses. Carers could ignore complications and merely reinforce the doctor's prescriptions, convinced that this is what is best. Meanwhile patients could sit back and take any hardships, firm in the knowledge that they are doing as they are told.

If we are truthful, we must all admit that we are making the best balances we can under challenging circumstances, recognise the desire to revert back to the traditional framework, but try to resist it and take responsibility for our own balances. Nobody said that this would be easy. The good news is that since our lives are so full of complexity and complex situations, we are already experts in complexity. It is just a matter of recognising and embracing this complexity so that reasonable outcomes can then come about. This expertise that patients and carers hold is being increasingly recognised by national administrations. For example, the UK government has recently established the 'Expert Patient Programme', a layperson-led educational intervention aimed at people living with a range of chronic diseases, diabetes among them (further details can be found at www.expertpatient.nhs.uk). Success here is down to people sharing their knowledge, their skills and their experiences with each other – in other words, peer mentorship!

Letting go of the fear and uncertainty and 'feeling yourself better'

As with many other chronic illnesses, the perception of the disease may be as crippling as the disease itself. Anxiety, depression and fear can gnaw at the mental and physical health of the patient, the carer and even the health professional. Unfortunately, in the UK, provision for supportive mental healthcare is sadly lacking, and mental healthcare is often stigmatised by society as being only for those who are 'crazy.' The problem is that the traditional orderly perspective tends to separate mind and body, the body being the embodiment of the mechanical, while the mind is more nebulous and uncertain. The result is that not only are mental and physical healthcare divided into different disciplines, but they are often physically separated in different buildings. For healthcare professionals, this means that so long as the physical aspects are all right, the mental state of the patient really isn't their problem. Or, if it does seem to be affecting the patient's physical condition, then the answer is to refer them to a different expert or prescribe some antidepressants and hope that the problem goes away. For the carer, it is a matter of finding a new expert to tell him or her what to do. For the patient, it can be very frightening. Not only is the body malfunctioning, but the mind is going as well!

Complexity can't solve this problem. However, unlike the traditional approach, it does recognise the importance of the interwoven physical and mental aspects of diabetes. It argues that if one is going to effectively support people with diabetes, the health system must pay more attention to, and spend more money on, mental health aspects. Similarly, complementary therapies that have been shown to have an impact on mental health must be rigorously researched to support their common use in medical practice. These may be as simple as the relaxation exercises outlined in the preceding chapter, or as skilled as acupuncture or homeopathy. Even more important than this is the role of the carers and patients themselves. From a complexity perspective, they are making key health decisions every day of the week. Recognising that they are important and that they make a difference can be a remarkably powerful 'cure' for overcoming the fear of diabetes or other chronic illnesses. Similarly, realising that diabetes is just another part of a complex system that they need to adapt to, and that they are already complexity experts – as they have already learned how to adapt to other situations in life – may be key to helping them to let go of the fear and uncertainty.

From this perspective, diabetes can be transformed from being a 'frozen accident' where new constraints are locked into place (diet, insulin, etc.) to a 'gateway event' where new possibilities emerge (greater self-awareness, new focus on life, etc.). In this case, diabetes can become a doorway to 'feeling yourself better.' The key for patients, carers and health professionals is to move out of the traditional framework, to recognise the possibility and power of self-learning, and to slowly work towards it.

Little steps may be just as important as big ones

As we discussed in Chapter 2, one of the best-known concepts from complexity theory is the 'butterfly effect' (Hollywood even made a bad movie about it!). A butterfly flapping its wings in China may trigger a tornado in Canada – the proverbial straw that breaks the camel's back, or snowflake that starts the avalanche. If we stop and think about it, tiny events are always having major impacts on our lives. A chance meeting, a missed bus or a forgotten meal can all have major outcomes. At the same time, thousands if not millions of small events pass by without any significant effect. Not every butterfly matters!

With diabetes, the big steps are always important – good diet, reasonable exercise, proper usage of medication and good communication between patient, carers and health professionals. However, little things can also be important tipping points for loss of blood glucose control. A stressful situation, forgotten insulin, and miscommunication between patient and GP can all trigger significant problems. Thankfully, most of these little steps pass by almost unnoticed or are contained within the normal boundaries of the more fundamental 'big steps.'

So what does this teach us? First, patients, carers and health professionals can't just follow core guidelines and expect them to work all of the time. Most people know this as 'common sense', but some (often basing their thinking on the traditional approach) desperately try to act otherwise. The patient and carer struggling to do as they are told, and the GP rigidly following the latest 'best practice', are all caught by the same logic. This does not mean that basic guidelines are not correct. It just forces us to recognise that uncertainties are always there, no matter how hard we try to follow the correct procedure – blood glucose levels, as we all know, do not always follow a recognised path.

Secondly, be aware of the little steps and try to learn from them, but realise that new ones will always surprise you. Imagine a person with type 1 diabetes (we'll call her Jessie) who has a minor car accident. While driving to the shops, she backs into a parked vehicle. No one is injured, and damage to the car is minor, but the other driver calls the police. Unfortunately, while she is waiting for the police to arrive, Jessie starts to feel 'hypo' and suddenly realises that she has no glucose sweets or snacks with her.

She starts to panic just as the police arrive. The police response is to take her to the hospital! Later, she reviews the episode and concludes that she will never leave the house without glucose sweets and a carbohydrate snack again! She has learned a valuable lesson. Next time, a different problem will strike and she will have to reassess her strategies once more.

Getting your daily dose of learning: the strengths and limits of knowledge, and the knowledge of strengths and limits

As complexity in general and the butterfly effect in particular demonstrate, with complex systems you never stop learning. New situations are constantly emerging and new combinations of events are continually creating different outcomes. Learning in this sense is much more than just memorisation. The traditional approach to learning was fundamentally repetitive and based on memory and hierarchies of knowledge. Those above you know more than you do – repeat and memorise what they do, and if you work hard enough you can eventually rise to the top of the knowledge tree. Universities and hospitals with their departments and specialisms still function predominantly along these lines.

From a complexity approach, learning is much more than memorisation. It is a continual process of exploration of the strengths and limits of knowledge. Going back to our box diagrams in Chapter 2, learning is about getting a feel for where certain phenomena belong in the orderly, complex or disorderly boxes, and recognising where certainty and predictability apply and where they do not. Fundamentally, learning from a complexity perspective isn't about accumulating a stack of knowledge, but about constantly exploring the strengths and limits of knowledge. For the health professional, this means being aware of the latest research on diabetes, but also shaping that knowledge to fit the unique and distinctive needs of each particular patient. It means having not only the confidence to offer 'best practice' to your patients, but also the courage to help them to make health choices that may fall outside these practices – not an easy thing to do when the entire thrust of government policy is on adherence to the guidelines and accountability to centralised criteria! One well-known researcher, Trisha Greenhalgh, summarised this conundrum very neatly when she described the difficulties of 'Narrative-based medicine in an evidence-based world.'[1]

For carers, it is about balancing the broader knowledge of health professionals with your detailed and intimate knowledge of the patient, and learning from both sides. If you look back at the Stacey diagram in Chapter 5, you will quickly see that carers are caught in a very complex position. As they lack technical knowledge, it is difficult for them to make judgements on complicated technical matters (zone 2). Also, being carers, they can never know exactly what the patient really wants. Thus they can never be completely certain about the 'political' personal aspects of the patient (zone 3). Slavishly doing as they are told by the health professionals is not the role of a carer from a complexity perspective. Likewise, stubbornly refusing the advice of professionals is equally distorting. Carers are caught in the zone of complexity (zone 4) and must constantly balance the aspects of both sides against each other. This is never easy, and requires continual learning and adaptation from both sides. The importance of this type of carer learning is recognised by health professionals, but resources to support carers remain woefully inadequate. Learning from the experience of other carers is one of the most powerful tools and, as we mentioned previously, this is now being absorbed into the Expert Patient Programme.

For patients, the focus is on combining their inherent personal knowledge with the technical knowledge of the health professional (and possibly with that of a carer). The health professional will dominate zones 1 and 2, but the patient is the expert in zone 3. Yes, they can work with the health professional and use their technical expertise, but they should realise that this will only take them so far. As soon as the patient leaves the health professional's office, a world of complexity situations will hit them. And even if they had a doctor continually by their side giving them expert advice, there are plenty of areas where the experts are often in disagreement, and all kinds of complex situations (zones 4 and 5) where they would only be able to give partial advice, or advice based purely on intuition at best. For patients coming from a traditional approach where patient passivity was the primary value, recognising their personal importance and responsibility for their own health outcomes can be a major challenge. However, if they have the courage to confront that challenge, the rewards can be huge.

Is there such a thing as a 'final cure' for diabetes?

There are encouraging developments in a number of fields for the treatment of diabetes. Insulin inhalers are now available, transplantation of pancreatic islet cells has been performed successfully, stem-cell therapy may be round the corner, insulin pumps, non-invasive glucose-monitoring systems (no needles!) and probably some sort of vaccine will be available within the next 10 years to prevent type 1 diabetes. Some of these developments may significantly ease the burden of diabetes, particularly type 1 diabetes, and could reduce complications, but will they provide a 'final cure' for diabetes and improve overall health? From a traditional perspective, it must be better. Improved treatments automatically lead to fewer complications, resulting in better health. Given enough time, effort and improved treatments, a final cure may be found, another disease ticked off the list and overall health will improve. Once this cure has been found, it is only a matter of spreading the treatment around the world. The eradication of smallpox is the classic case.

It is a much more difficult question to answer from a complexity perspective. For example, the vast majority of diabetes is type 2, and this is often brought on by lifestyle choices (particularly in wealthy countries), such as poor diet, obesity and minimal exercise. Even if better, more convenient and more effective treatments become available, this could easily lead to an increase, not a decrease, in complications. If type 2 diabetes could be simply dealt with by an easy squirt from an inhaler, then why bother to change one's life at all? Individuals would merely continue their poor eating and exercising habits, and other types of illness/disease would accelerate.

From a complexity perspective, a 'final cure' for diabetes is at best a mixed blessing. Yes, for many individuals with type 1 diabetes some form of cure would be a tremendous benefit, enabling them to live possibly longer and healthier lives. However, as discussed above, for many others (particularly with type 2), diabetes is merely a symptom of the accumulation of underlying negative lifestyle choices. 'Curing' diabetes without addressing these underlying causes may actually worsen the prevailing epidemic and result in negative health outcomes overall. Basically, complex chronic illnesses are really mirrors of the complex nature of life. And what is life but a continual balancing of physical, chemical and biological processes interwoven with the complex social norms and choices that pervade our societies and individual lives? Diabetes and other chronic illnesses complicate this balancing act but do not alter it fundamentally. There is no final stable point of perfect health or, for that matter, of endless life (the ultimate dream of perfect health). Life is complexity, not order.

Complexity is the norm: learn to recognise and accept it in diabetes and elsewhere

As we have argued throughout this book, we believe that there is a fundamental shift taking place in science, medicine and health – a shift from order to complexity. This doesn't mean that everything is getting more complex (although in many ways it is), but rather that we are just beginning to recognise the importance and power of complexity in our surroundings and daily lives. Diabetes is just one aspect of this overall complexity. For much of the twentieth century, the problem hasn't been complexity, but our desperate desire to find some sort of fixed order in our societies, politics and health. Whether this is a dictator imposing his vision of 'final order' on a cowed populace, or a doctor imprisoning diabetic patients because they could not be trusted to follow their prescribed diets and medication, the logic is the same. Some of the major horrors of the twentieth century can be blamed on the pursuit of 'final order.'

Complexity isn't a problem for those who can embrace it. Complexity is a normal aspect of life – wonderful, challenging and surprising, but also threatening, discouraging and uncertain. Diabetes and its management are no different. Even if we could find a final cure, new health challenges would emerge to take its place. This is not a call for complacency or for giving up, but a recognition of the ongoing centrality of complexity in our lives and the danger of a false belief in the power of 'order' to bring about a final solution to our problems. In a small way, we hope that this book will help you to embrace the complexity of diabetes as a patient, carer or health practitioner.

One more point – complexity does not end with diabetes. As we have learned from our students and patients, once you begin to view the world from a complexity perspective it is difficult to stop. Daily routines, common interactions, personal relationships, job developments, organisational structures, life choices . . . you name it and complexity thinking has implications for it. Where will this lead you? At an intellectual and societal level, there are growing signs of the spread of complexity thinking in virtually every major academic discipline and policy arena. Often policy actors are speaking the language of complexity without knowing it. For them, recognising complexity is tantamount to admitting defeat. *Hopefully, this book has convinced you that rather than representing defeat, recognising complexity is the first step towards a greater understanding of the real world around us.* At a personal level, the ways in which the recognition of complexity and its tools will affect your life, only you can know! Just start exploring and don't be afraid. Mistakes, failure and meandering along your own personal fitness landscape are all part of the process. As the quote from the Stereophonics at the beginning of this chapter says, 'you gotta go there to come back'!

If you are convinced, reflect and do

Our final lesson is a simple and short one – if you are convinced, reflect and do. For us, complexity is the science of pragmatism and 'common sense.' Everyone knows that life and diabetes are complex. However, time after time, simple orderly mechanical frameworks for diabetes and health keep reappearing. Whether they are politicians determined to show that they are 'in control' of the health system, drug companies who claim to have 'cured' a common illness, or individuals believing that more 'order' in their lives would make things better, the desire for final 'orders' infects our health and social systems.

The real problem for the complexity approach is that it promises so little. There is no final happy place for complexity, there are no final health solutions, and we are all (to some degree) responsible for our own health outcomes. Moreover, the most exciting rallying cry that complexity can offer is '*Be balanced.*' Nevertheless, what complexity can do for you as a patient, carer and/or health professional is help you to realise that the diabetes rollercoaster is normal and a mirror of life itself. There are always smooth bits and rough bits, and anyone who says that they can make it a nice easy ride is, as the old saying goes, 'either lying or trying to sell you something.' In the end, it is what you make of the ride that really matters.

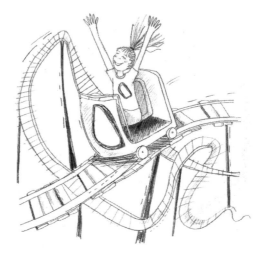

Reference

1   Greenhalgh T. Narrative-based medicine in an evidence-based world. *BMJ.* 1999; **318**: 323–5.

Index

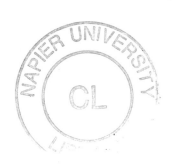